New Advances in Hip and Knee Reconstructive Surgery

New Advances in Hip and Knee Reconstructive Surgery

Guest Editor
Senthil Sambandam

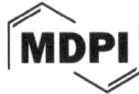

Basel • Beijing • Wuhan • Barcelona • Belgrade • Novi Sad • Cluj • Manchester

Guest Editor
Senthil Sambandam
Department of Orthopedics
University of Texas
Southwestern
Dallas, TX
USA

Editorial Office
MDPI AG
Grosspeteranlage 5
4052 Basel, Switzerland

This is a reprint of the Special Issue, published open access by the journal *Journal of Clinical Medicine* (ISSN 2077-0383), freely accessible at: https://www.mdpi.com/journal/jcm/special_issues/323L2BO51Z.

For citation purposes, cite each article independently as indicated on the article page online and as indicated below:

Lastname, A.A.; Lastname, B.B. Article Title. *Journal Name* **Year**, *Volume Number*, Page Range.

ISBN 978-3-7258-4283-4 (Hbk)
ISBN 978-3-7258-4284-1 (PDF)
https://doi.org/10.3390/books978-3-7258-4284-1

© 2025 by the authors. Articles in this book are Open Access and distributed under the Creative Commons Attribution (CC BY) license. The book as a whole is distributed by MDPI under the terms and conditions of the Creative Commons Attribution-NonCommercial-NoDerivs (CC BY-NC-ND) license (https://creativecommons.org/licenses/by-nc-nd/4.0/).

Contents

Killian Cosendey, Julien Stanovici, Hugues Cadas, Patrick Omoumi, Brigitte M. Jolles and Julien Favre
Simultaneous Evaluation of Bone Cut and Implant Placement Accuracy in Robotic-Assisted Total Knee Arthroplasty
Reprinted from: *J. Clin. Med.* **2024**, *13*, 1293, https://doi.org/10.3390/jcm13051293 1

Kyun-Ho Shin, Jin-Ho Kim and Seung-Beom Han
Greater Risk of Periprosthetic Joint Infection Associated with Prolonged Operative Time in Primary Total Knee Arthroplasty: Meta- Analysis of 427,361 Patients
Reprinted from: *J. Clin. Med.* **2024**, *13*, 3046, https://doi.org/10.3390/jcm13113046 13

Hunter B. Jones, Andrew J. Hinkle, Yida Liu and Senthil N. Sambandam
Multivariate Analysis of Risk Factors for In-Hospital Dislocation Following Primary Total Hip Arthroplasty
Reprinted from: *J. Clin. Med.* **2024**, *13*, 3456, https://doi.org/10.3390/jcm13123456 25

Catalina Baez, Robert MacDonell, Abtahi Tishad, Hernan A. Prieto, Emilie N. Miley, Justin T. Deen, et al.
Comparison of Five-Day vs. Fourteen-Day Incubation of Cultures for Diagnosis of Periprosthetic Joint Infection in Hip Arthroplasty
Reprinted from: *J. Clin. Med.* **2024**, *13*, 4467, https://doi.org/10.3390/jcm13154467 33

Tizian Heinz, Hristo Vasilev, Philip Mark Anderson, Ioannis Stratos, Axel Jakuscheit, Konstantin Horas, et al.
Functional Outcome after Direct Anterior Approach Total Hip Arthroplasty (DAA-THA) for Coxa Profunda and Protrusio Acetabuli—A Retrospective Study
Reprinted from: *J. Clin. Med.* **2024**, *13*, 4596, https://doi.org/10.3390/jcm13164596 44

Catalina Baez, Hernan A. Prieto, Abtahi Tishad, Terrie Vasilopoulos, Emilie N. Miley, Justin T. Deen, et al.
Local Infiltration Analgesia Is Superior to Regional Nerve Blocks for Total Hip Arthroplasty: Less Falls, Better Mobility, and Same-Day Discharge
Reprinted from: *J. Clin. Med.* **2024**, *13*, 4645, https://doi.org/10.3390/jcm13164645 56

Anubhav Thapaliya, Mehul M. Mittal, Terrul L. Ratcliff, Varatharaj Mounasamy, Dane K. Wukich and Senthil N. Sambandam
Usage of Tranexamic Acid for Total Hip Arthroplasty: A Matched Cohort Analysis of 144,344 Patients
Reprinted from: *J. Clin. Med.* **2024**, *13*, 4920, https://doi.org/10.3390/jcm13164920 68

Peter Richard Almeida, Gavin J. Macpherson, Philip Simpson, Paul Gaston and Nick D. Clement
The Use of Highly Porous 3-D-Printed Titanium Acetabular Cups in Revision Total Hip Arthroplasty: A Systematic Review and Meta-Analysis
Reprinted from: *J. Clin. Med.* **2025**, *14*, 938, https://doi.org/10.3390/jcm14030938 78

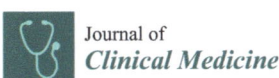

Article

Simultaneous Evaluation of Bone Cut and Implant Placement Accuracy in Robotic-Assisted Total Knee Arthroplasty

Killian Cosendey [1], Julien Stanovici [1], Hugues Cadas [2], Patrick Omoumi [3], Brigitte M. Jolles [1,4] and Julien Favre [1,5,*]

1. Department of Musculoskeletal Medicine, Lausanne University Hospital and University of Lausanne (CHUV-UNIL), CH-1011 Lausanne, Switzerland; killian.cosendey@chuv.ch (K.C.); brigitte.jolles-haeberli@chuv.ch (B.M.J.)
2. Morphology and Anatomy Faculty Unit, University of Lausanne (UNIL), CH-1005 Lausanne, Switzerland; hugues.cadas@unil.ch
3. Department of Diagnostic and Interventional Radiology, Lausanne University Hospital and University of Lausanne (CHUV-UNIL), CH-1011 Lausanne, Switzerland; patrick.omoumi@chuv.ch
4. Institute of Electrical and Micro Engineering, Ecole Polytechnique Fédérale de Lausanne (EPFL), CH-1015 Lausanne, Switzerland
5. The Sense Innovation and Research Center, CH-1007 Lausanne, Switzerland
* Correspondence: julien.favre@chuv.ch

Abstract: Background: This study aimed to evaluate the accuracy of bone cuts and implant placements, simultaneously, for total knee arthroplasty (TKA) performed using a system with an active robotic arm. **Methods:** Two experienced orthopaedic surgeons performed TKA on ten cadaveric legs. Computed tomography scans were performed to compare the bone cuts and implant placements with the preoperative planning. The differences between the planned and actual bone cuts and implant placements were assessed using positional and angular errors in the three anatomical planes. Additionally, the cut–implant deviations were calculated. Statistical analysis was performed to detect systematic errors in the bone cuts and implant placements and to quantify the correlations between these errors. **Results:** The root-mean-square (RMS) errors of the bone cuts (with respect to the planning) were between 0.7–1.5 mm and 0.6–1.7°. The RMS implant placement errors (with respect to the planning) varied between 0.6–1.6 mm and 0.4–1.5°, except for the femur and tibia in the sagittal plane (2.9°). Systematic errors in the bone cuts and implant placements were observed, respectively, in three and two degrees of freedom. For cut–implant deviations, the RMS values ranged between 0.3–2.0 mm and 0.6–1.9°. The bone cut and implant placement errors were significantly correlated in eight degrees-of-freedom ($\rho \geq 0.67$, $p < 0.05$). **Conclusions:** With most of the errors below 2 mm or 2°, this study supported the value of active robotic TKA in achieving accurate bone cuts and implant placements. The findings also highlighted the need for both accurate bone cuts and proper implantation technique to achieve accurate implant placements.

Keywords: total knee arthroplasty; robotic-assisted surgery; accuracy; bone cuts and implant placements; position and orientation errors

1. Introduction

Robotic assistance is very promising in total knee arthroplasty (TKA), specifically to achieve accurate bone cuts and thus increase the accuracy of implant placements. This is particularly important because a more accurate placement of implants has been suggested to improve patient-reported outcomes [1–3]. Such benefits, in comparison to conventional surgery, have already been reported with some robotic-assisted systems, notably improvements in implant placement accuracy, increases in patient satisfaction, and/or reductions in complications [3,4]. Nevertheless, not all robotic systems are necessarily equally effective. Therefore, there is a need to assess the systems and their new releases continuously to ensure that they are used properly and possibly also to highlight areas of improvement.

Over the years, diverse approaches to TKA robotic assistance have been proposed, some moving surgical tools and others monitoring the movement of the surgical tools moved by the surgeons. Differences also exist in the means of cutting the bone, with some solutions using a saw and others using a cutter. One interesting option is the TSOLUTION ONE® Total Knee Application ("TSOLUTION ONE" in this article, THINK Surgical Inc., Fremont, CA, USA). It includes a surgery device with a robotic arm controlling a cutter (named TCAT®) and a surgical planning workstation (named TPLAN®). It differentiates itself from the other options currently on the market by the fact that it is the only system that actively cuts the bones. So far, this system has been reported to cut the bones with root-mean-square errors below 2 mm and 1° in six degrees of freedom for both the femur and the tibia [5]. The root-mean-square errors in implant placements within 1.5 mm and 1.5° have also been reported for eight degrees of freedom, including the femoral anterior–posterior position and internal–external rotation angle, as well as the femoral and tibial proximal–distal position, flexion–extension and varus–valgus angles [6]. While these previous studies provide important insights, they differ on several aspects, which prevents the combination of their results, for example, to assess the deviations between the bone cuts and the implant placements. Indeed, in addition to differences in implant types and error calculation methods, one study analysed implant placements in human knees [6], whereas another assessed bone cuts using sawbone knees [5]. Consequently, additional studies simultaneously assessing the accuracy of bone cuts and the accuracy of implant placements are needed for the TSOLUTION ONE system. Evaluating the deviations between bone cuts and implant placements is particularly motivated by previous studies on manual TKA, showing that implants are not always placed perfectly in contact with the cut surfaces of bones [7–9] and by the fact that the deviations could be different with bones cut by a robotic arm rather than manually.

The purpose of this study was to assess the accuracy of bone cuts and implant placements simultaneously for TKA performed using the TSOLUTION ONE system. The study also aimed to evaluate the cut–implant deviations.

2. Materials and Methods

Following approval from the local ethics committee, TKA was performed on 10 formalin-fixed, anonymized cadaveric legs using the TSOLUTION ONE system (version 300). The sample size was determined based on previous comparable studies and ethical considerations [10–12]. According to local regulations regarding research on deceased persons, no demographic data were available for the samples. The procedures were performed by two senior orthopaedic surgeons from our university hospital, with more than 5 years of independent TKA practice. The surgeons, who were previously trained on the system using sawbones and cadaveric knees, conducted, respectively, four and six cases, following the manufacturer's recommendations for regular TKA on patients. To increase reliability, all data acquisition and processing were conducted by a single operator [13]. The 6-step protocol used for each study knee is described below.

Step 1: five fiducial markers (titanium beads of 0.8 mm diameter) were embedded in the femur and tibia to allow them to register the original bones (before cutting) with the cut bones in step 4.

Step 2: Preoperative CT images of the cadaveric leg were acquired with a Discovery CT750 HD machine (GE Healthcare, Chicago, IL, USA) parametrised as follows: field of view of 250 × 250 mm, matrix size of 512 × 512 pixels, tube voltage of 120 kVp and tube current of 200 mAs. Two different slice thicknesses were used: high resolution of 0.312 mm and low resolution of 0.625 mm. After uploading the low-resolution CT images in the surgical planning software, the three-dimensional (3D) surface models of the bones were reconstructed and used to plan the TKA. For this study, all procedures were carried out with the "Unity Posterior Stabilized Femoral" implant and the "Unity Tibial" implant (Corin, Cirencester, UK). Once the planning was completed by the surgeon, it was transferred to the robotic device.

Step 3: The preparation and calibration of the robot followed the standard procedure of any TKA intervention on patients. Next, the surgeon exposed the cadaveric knee following a medial parapatellar approach. Following the instructions on the robot's screen, the surgeon then recorded the position of registration points on the surface of the bones using a mechanical digitizer. After that, the robot registered the 3D surface model of the bones on the actual bones and cut the femoral and tibial bones according to the planning (Figure 1). The bones were cut autonomously by the robot, under the surgeon's supervision. Once the bone cuts were completed, nylon implants were impacted and cemented by the surgeon who then sutured the leg following the usual procedure. Nylon implants were used to avoid the artefacts in the CT images induced by the metal of regular implants particularly affecting the bone (cut) close to the implants [14,15].

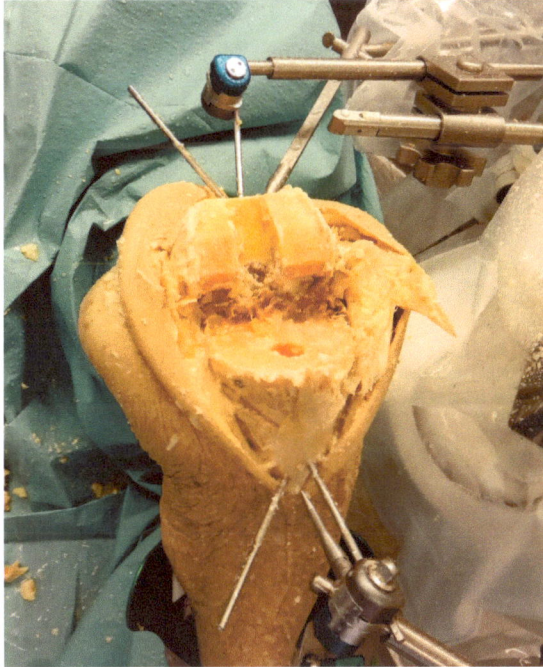

Figure 1. Example of a study knee after bone cutting.

Step 4: Postoperative CT images of the cadaveric leg were acquired using the same high-resolution parameters as for the preoperative CT scan described in step 2. Based on these images, the 3D surface models of the cut bones and of the implants were reconstructed using in-house software. Then, the cut bone models and the implant models were imported in the preoperative CT frame and registered on the preoperative data (original bone models and planning). Registrations were carried out separately for the tibia and the femur by locating the centre of the fiducial markers and calculating the mathematical transformation, mapping the markers of the cut bones to the markers of the original bones [16].

Step 5: To quantify the accuracy, cut and implant frames using the same definition as the planning frames were embedded in the 3D surface models of the cut bones and in the 3D surface models of the implants. Then, the differences between the planning frames and the cut frames as well as between the planning frames and the implant frames were calculated as three positional and three angular errors. The errors were expressed in the anatomical frames proposed by Victor et al. [17]. Additionally, the cut–implant deviations, defined as the difference between the implant placement errors and the bone cut errors, were calculated independently for each degree of freedom. By convention, positive femoral errors indicate a cut or an implant too lateral, proximal, anterior, varus, internally rotated and extended compared to the planning or compared to the cut. Tibial errors were defined similarly to the femoral errors, except in the coronal and sagittal planes, where positives errors indicate a cut or an implant too flexed and valgus compared to the planning or compared to the cut. Since the internal–external rotation of the tibia implant was not constrained by the bone cuts, no error was calculated for this degree of freedom.

To assess the reliability of the error measurement method, two randomly selected knees were CT-scanned and processed five times each by the single operator in this study. This procedure indicated root-mean-square (RMS) differences among repeats under 0.2 mm and 0.3° for all positional and angular errors.

Statistical Analysis

Bone cut errors, implant placement errors and cut–implant deviations were reported through their median, interquartile range (IQR) and root-mean-square (RMS). In adequacy with a study population limited to 10 knees, data were tested using non-parametric statistics. Specifically, systematic errors (i.e., biases) were detected using Kruskal–Wallis tests, followed by post hoc Wilcoxon signed-rank tests with Bonferroni corrections. Spearman's rho correlations were calculated between bone cut and implant placement errors to estimate the influence of the bone cut errors on the implant placement errors. The significance level was set a priori to 5%. In addition, the number of knees presenting outlier errors or deviations (defined as errors or deviations exceeding ± 3 mm or ± 3°) was recorded [18]. Data processing and statistical analysis were performed with Matlab R2019b (Mathworks, Natick, MA, USA).

3. Results

Errors and deviations are reported using boxplots in Figures 2 and 3, whereas numbers are provided in Appendix A (Tables A1 and A2).

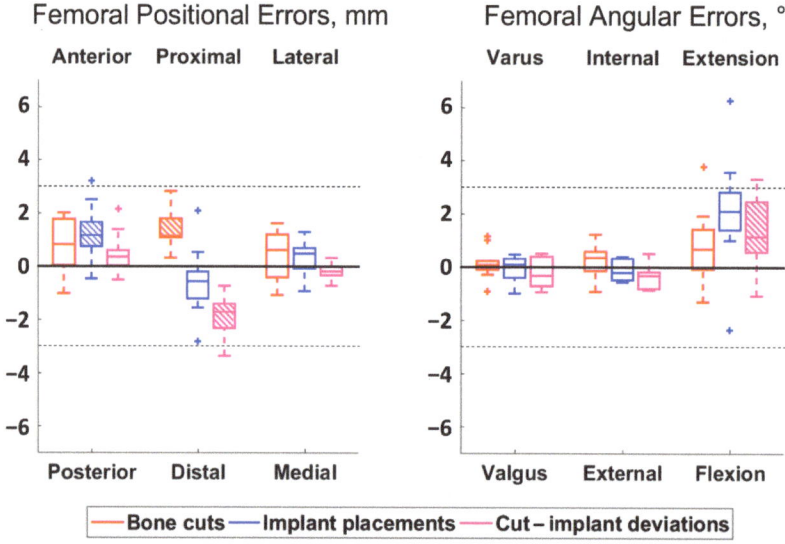

Figure 2. Boxplot of the positional (**left**) and angular (**right**) errors and deviations for the femur. Each boxplot displays the interquartile range (box), median value (line), and outliers (crosses). The directions above and below the plots indicate where the actual cuts or implant placements were compared to the planning or compared to the cuts. Hatched boxes indicate errors or deviations statistically significantly different from zero (i.e., with a bias) (adjusted $p < 0.05$). Dashed lines are included at ±3 mm and ±3° to delineate the outlier thresholds.

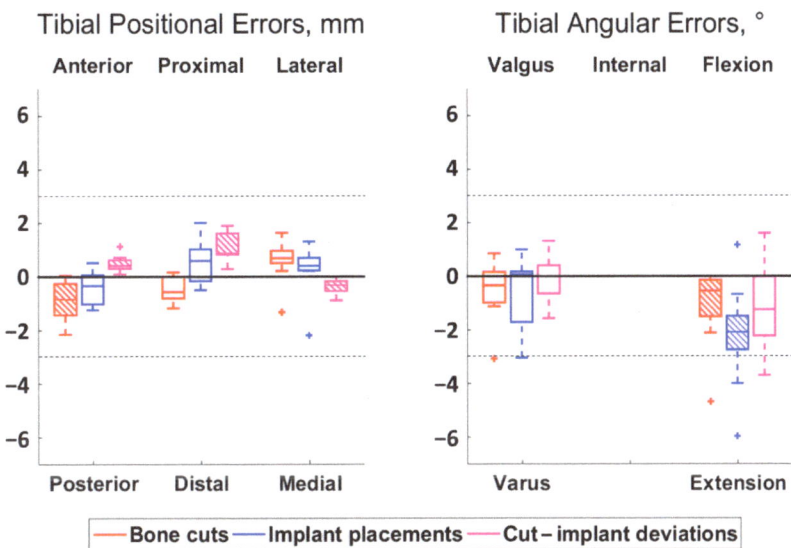

Figure 3. Boxplot of the positional (**left**) and angular (**right**) errors and deviations for the tibia. Each boxplot displays the interquartile range (box), median value (line), and outliers (crosses). The directions above and below the plots indicate where the actual cuts or implant placements were compared to the planning or compared to the cuts. Hatched boxes indicate errors or deviations statistically significantly different from zero (i.e., with a bias) (adjusted $p < 0.05$). Dashed lines are included at ± 3 mm and $\pm 3°$ to delineate the outlier thresholds.

Regarding the bone cut errors, the RMS values ranged between 0.7–1.5 mm and 0.6–1.7°. Three cases of bias were observed: in the femoral proximal–distal position ($p = 0.01$), with cuts too proximal compared to the planning (median error of 1.2 mm), and in the tibial antero–posterior position ($p = 0.01$) and flexion–extension angle ($p = 0.01$), with cuts too posterior and extended compared to the planning (median errors of 0.8 mm and 0.5°, respectively). In total, 3 of the 110 individual measurements exceeded the ± 3 mm or 3° thresholds and were considered outliers.

The RMS errors of the implant placements varied between 0.6–1.6 mm and 0.4–1.5°, except in the femoral and tibial flexion–extension angles, where the errors had RMS values of 2.9°. Two cases of bias were observed: in the femoral anterior–posterior position ($p = 0.02$), with implants too anterior compared to the planning (median errors of 1.2 mm), and in the tibial flexion–extension angle ($p = 0.02$), with implants too extended compared to the planning (median errors of 2.1°). A total of 6 outlier errors were observed, from the 110 individual measurements.

Regarding the deviation between bone cuts and implant placements, the RMS values ranged between 0.3–2.0 mm and 0.6–1.9°. Five cases of bias were observed, as illustrated in Figure 4: in the femoral proximal–distal position ($p = 0.01$) and the flexion–extension angle ($p = 0.04$), with implants too distal and extended compared to the cuts (median differences of 1.7 mm and 1.2°, respectively), and in the tibial anterior–posterior ($p = 0.01$), proximal–distal ($p = 0.01$) and medio-lateral ($p = 0.01$) positions with implants too anterior, proximal and medial compared to the cuts (median differences of 0.4 mm, 0.9 mm and 0.3 mm, respectively). A total of 4 outlier deviations were observed out of the 110 individual measurements. Statistically significant correlations between implant placement errors and bone cut errors were observed for four out of the six degrees of freedom in the femur and for four out of the five degrees of freedom in the tibia ($\rho \geq 0.67$, $p < 0.05$) (Figures 5 and 6). The statistically non-significant correlations were in the femoral varus–

valgus angle ($p = 0.26$), in the femoral flexion–extension angle ($p = 0.07$) and in the tibial flexion–extension angle ($p = 0.97$).

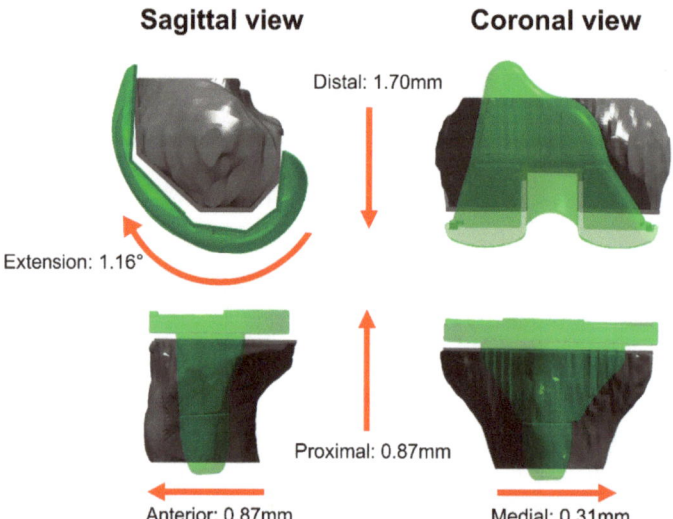

Figure 4. Illustration of the biases in cut–implant deviations for a right knee. The red arrows represent the systematic deviations (median values) observed on the 10 study knees.

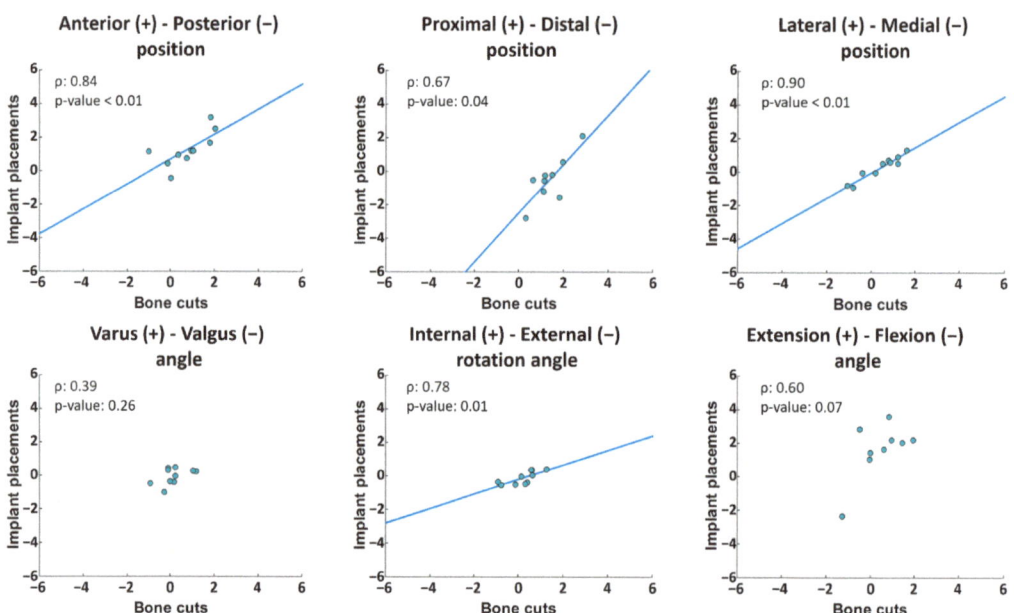

Figure 5. Correlations between femoral bone cut and implant placement errors. When the correlation was statistically significant, the linear regression line was plotted. Data are in mm for positional errors and in degree for angular errors. ρ: Spearman's rank coefficient of correlation.

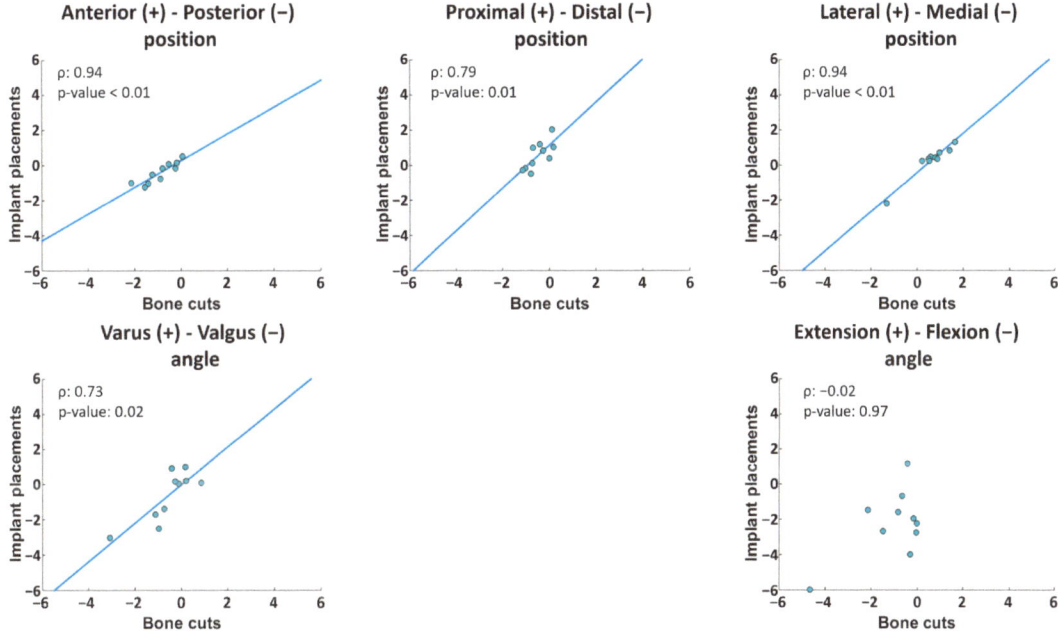

Figure 6. Correlations between tibial bone cut and implant placement errors. When the correlation was statistically significant, the linear regression line was plotted. Data are in mm for positional errors and in degree for angular errors. ρ: Spearman's rank coefficient of correlation.

4. Discussion

The results showed accurate bone cuts, with RMS errors below 2 mm or 2° and less than 3% outliers (3 out of 110 errors). These results are consistent with a previous study assessing the same system on sawbones [5]. In fact, the median errors differed by less than 0.6 mm or 0.8° between both studies that used distinctive experimental settings, suggesting that the bone cut errors reported in these two studies should indeed correspond to the real accuracy ranges of the system.

The accuracy of implant placements was in the same range as the bone cut accuracy for nine out of the eleven degrees of freedom (RMS errors under 2 mm or 2°, 2.2% of outliers). These results agreed with a prior study evaluating the same robotic system with patients [6]. In the two other degrees of freedom, femoral and tibial flexion–extension, the RMS errors were 2.9° with 20% outliers. This lower accuracy seemed attributable to the implantation process, since the accuracy of the bone cuts was not markedly lower in these two degrees of freedom than in the others. Interestingly, larger implant placement errors in flexion–extension were not reported in the prior study evaluating the TSOLUTION ONE system [6]. It is therefore possible that the cut–implant deviations vary among implant designs and/or implantation techniques. This possibility is supported by the literature, as other studies evaluating the angular accuracy of TKA performed with image-free navigation systems have also reported larger cut–implant deviations in the sagittal plane [7–9]. Further research assessing the error of bone cuts and of implant placements simultaneously, as in the present study, are thus notably encouraged to identify preferable prosthesis designs or implementation techniques.

A novelty of this study was to characterize the cut–implant deviations both in terms of positions and angles. Deviations between bone cuts and implant placements were generally low, with RMS errors below 2 mm or 2° and no outliers observed in eight of the eleven degrees of freedom. Furthermore, statistically significant correlations were found between bone cut and implant placement errors in seven of these eight degrees of freedom, highlighting the importance of accurate bone cuts for accurate implant placements. Nevertheless, outliers in the cut–implant deviations were observed for the remaining three degrees of freedom, specifically in the tibial flexion–extension angle (10% of outliers), consistent with the literature [7,9], as well as in the femoral proximal–distal position and the flexion–extension angle (20% and 10% of outliers, respectively), for which no data were found in the literature. The limited access to the posterior region of the knee due to the anterior surgical exposure could have contributed to these larger deviations, as the posterior aspect of the implants might have been more difficult to impact. Altogether, these results agree with previous studies which have reported that, despite accurate bone cuts, cement thickness and impaction can cause implant placement errors and induce malalignment [7,19,20]. Therefore, it appears essential to perform the implantation process with caution, particularly regarding the proximal–distal positions and flexion–extension angles. In the future, it might also be possible to reduce the cut–implant deviations by improving implant designs and implantation instrumentations.

Since biases were observed in this study, and it is noteworthy to wonder whether different command of the robotic device could limit them. Although theoretically possible (for example, the femoral bone could be cut more proximally to reduce the proximal–distal implant placement error), a better understanding of the sources of biases would be necessary to ensure that such modifications would actually be beneficial. Indeed, various factors could influence the biases, such as implants, registration points, or calibration of the robotic system, and modifying the command based on one situation could be harmful in other situations. Furthermore, the biases were relatively small and not the sole source of errors. For example, the biases accounted only for a portion of the outlier errors that were observed, up to 3.3 mm and 6.3°. Consequently, further investigations are necessary to understand the sources of both the biases and the outliers. Clarifying this could suggest ways to reduce the bone cut and implant placement errors by acting on the robot or on another aspect of TKA.

Compiling data from two systematic reviews on the accuracy of robotic-assisted systems [21,22] enabled the identification of five cadaveric studies with variables of interest similar to those investigated in the present study [10–12,23,24]. Of course, the results in all these studies cannot be rigorously compared, due to variations in experimental aspects (e.g., robotic approach, number and condition of the knees, and assessment methods), and it was not an objective of the present study to compare systems. Nevertheless, it is interesting to put side by side all these results, keeping in mind the variations in experimental aspects. Doing so suggested quite consistent results among the studies, with mean or median errors ranging from 0.0° to 1.3° for femoral and tibial bone cut accuracy (current study: 0.1° to 0.8°) and mean or median errors ranging from 0.1° to 2.0° for femoral and tibial implant placement (current study: 0.1° to 2.1°). Consequently, the current results and those from prior studies, support the potential of robotic-assisted systems for accurate bone cuts and implant placements in TKA.

Several limitations of the present study should be outlined. First, the implants used in this study were nylon, a material that differs structurally from conventional implants, and this could have affected the implantation procedures. However, the use of nylon implants reduced the artefacts in CT scans, enabling more accurate measurement of bone cuts and implant placements. Second, the use of cadaveric specimens led to different bone quality and reduced the mental pressure compared to TKA performed on patients, which could influence the results. Nonetheless, the use of cadaveric samples allowed for the insertion of metallic beads in the bones and the use of nylon implants, which contributed to more accurate assessments. Third, only one type of implant was used. A different prosthesis model could yield different results mainly for implant placement errors and cut–implant deviations. Therefore, further research will be necessary to evaluate the possibility of generalizing the findings to other types of implants. Lastly, the sample size was small, and limited information was available concerning the cadaveric specimens due to ethical and regulatory considerations. A larger population, with an extensive characterization of the specimens, for example, including demographic or structural data, could allow for more specific assessment of the errors and methods, thus highlighting possible areas of improvement. Including a wider panel of surgeons and a control group with conventional surgery could also contribute to a deeper understanding. While these perspectives are attractive, it is noteworthy that the study protocol was adapted to the present objectives and consistent with previous cadaveric studies assessing bone cut and implant placement errors in TKA [10–12,23].

5. Conclusions

This study confirmed the capacity of the TSOLUTION ONE system to achieve accurate bone cuts, both in terms of positions and angles. Moreover, the implant placement accuracy was in the same range as the bone cut accuracy, except in the femoral and tibial flexion–extension angles. This decrease in accuracy could be due to the implantation process, which was the only step occurring between bone cuts and implant placements. Another notable finding of this study concerns the cut–implant deviations, which indicated that accurate bone cuts were necessary for accurate implant placements. But this was not enough; the results also highlighted the importance of the implantation and the possibilities to improve the accuracy of the implant placements by acting on factors such as cement thickness, impaction, or knee exposure. While this study confirmed that robotic-assisted systems can achieve accurate bone cuts and implant placements in TKA, further studies will be required to determine the relationships between these accuracies and the clinical outcomes.

Author Contributions: Conceptualisation, K.C., J.S., H.C., P.O., B.M.J. and J.F.; data curation, K.C.; formal analysis, K.C.; funding acquisition, B.M.J. and J.F.; investigation, K.C., J.S., H.C., P.O., B.M.J. and J.F.; methodology, K.C. and J.F.; project administration, K.C., P.O., B.M.J. and J.F.; resources, K.C., J.S., H.C., P.O., B.M.J. and J.F.; software, K.C. and J.F.; supervision, B.M.J. and J.F.; validation, K.C. and J.F.; visualisation, K.C.; writing—original draft, K.C. and J.F.; writing—review and editing, K.C., J.S., H.C., P.O., B.M.J. and J.F.; B.M.J. and J.F. supervised this study and should be considered as the last authors. All authors have read and agreed to the published version of the manuscript.

Funding: This research was partially funded by Think Surgical Inc. (Fremont, CA, USA).

Institutional Review Board Statement: The study was conducted in accordance with the Declaration of Helsinki, and approved by the ethics committee Vaud, Switzerland on August 9, 2019 (CER-VD 2019-01102).

Informed Consent Statement: Not applicable.

Data Availability Statement: The data are not publicly available due to regulatory provisions.

Acknowledgments: The authors would like to thank Christel Elandoy for her assistance in CT scanning.

Conflicts of Interest: The study was designed in consultation with Think Surgical Inc. and partially funded by Think Surgical. Data acquisition and analysis, as well as reporting were done independently by the authors. To avoid public disclosure of confidential information, Think Surgical Inc. had the opportunity to review the manuscript before its submission for publication.

Appendix A

Table A1. Positional and angular errors as well as deviations for the femur ($n = 10$ knees).

	Anterior (+)–posterior (−) position	Proximal (+)–distal (−) position	Lateral (+)–medial (−) position	Varus (+)–valgus (−) angle	Internal (+)–external (−) rotation angle	Extension (+)–flexion (−) angle
Bone cut errors						
Median [IQR]	0.84 [1.47]	1.16 [0.62] *	0.64 [1.37]	0.08 [0.33]	0.37 [0.66]	0.71 [1.37]
RMS	1.19	1.52	0.96	0.58	0.66	1.55
Percentage of outliers (%)	0	0	0	0	0	10
Implant placement errors						
Median [IQR]	1.17 [0.73] *	−0.55 [0.83]	0.50 [0.73]	0.10 [0.70]	−0.20 [0.72]	2.12 [1.21]
RMS	1.60	1.32	0.73	0.46	0.39	2.92
Percentage of outliers (%)	10	0	0	0	0	20
Cut–implant deviations						
Median [IQR]	0.37 [0.53]	−1.70 [0.75] *	−0.18 [0.29]	−0.31 [1.04]	−0.31 [0.57]	1.16 [1.52] *
RMS	0.89	2.02	0.32	0.56	0.55	1.80
Percentage of outliers (%)	0	20	0	0	0	10
ρ (p-value)	0.84 (<0.01)	0.67 (0.04)	0.90 (<0.01)	0.39 (0.26)	0.78 (0.01)	0.60 (0.07)

The values in this table indicate where the bone cuts or implant placements were compared to the planning or compared to the bone cuts. For example, a positive anterior–posterior error indicates an implant that was too anterior compared to the planning; similarly a negative varus–valgus deviation indicates an implant that was too valgus compared to the cut. Median, IQR and RMS data are in mm for positional errors and deviations and in degree for angular errors and deviations. IQR: interquartile range; RMS: root-mean-square; ρ: Spearman's rank coefficient of correlation. *: Statistically significantly different from zero ($p \leq 0.05$).

Table A2. Positional and angular errors as well as deviations for the tibia ($n = 10$ knees).

	Anterior (+)–posterior (−) position	Proximal (+)–distal (−) position	Lateral (+)–medial (−) position	Valgus (+)–varus (−) angle	Flexion (+)–extension (−) angle
Bone cut errors					
Median [IQR]	−0.83 [1.03] *	−0.56 [0.72]	0.69 [0.43]	−0.33 [1.01]	−0.54 [1.14] *
RMS	1.10	0.66	0.99	1.15	1.73
Percentage of outliers (%)	0	0	0	10	10

Table A2. Cont.

	Tibia				
	Anterior (+)–posterior (−) position	Proximal (+)–distal (−) position	Lateral (+)–medial (−) position	Valgus (+)–varus (−) angle	Flexion (+)–extension (−) angle
Implant placement errors					
Median [IQR]	−0.33 [0.96]	0.60 [1.12]	0.41 [0.39]	0.07 [1.80]	−2.09 [1.22] *
RMS	0.69	0.94	0.93	1.49	2.86
Percentage of outliers (%)	0	0	0	10	20
Cut–implant deviations					
Median [IQR]	0.43 [0.30] *	0.87 [0.64] *	−0.31 [0.28] *	0.00 [0.98]	−1.24 [1.91]
RMS	0.56	1.16	0.42	0.80	1.89
Percentage of outliers (%)	0	0	0	0	10
ρ (p-value)	0.94 (<0.01)	0.79 (0.01)	0.94 (<0.01)	0.73 (0.02)	−0.02 (0.97)

The values in this table indicate where the bone cuts or implant placements were compared to the planning or the bone cuts. For example, a negative anterior-posterior error indicates an implant that was too posterior compared to the planning, similarly a positive proximal–distal deviation indicates an implant that was too proximal compared to the cut. Median, IQR and RMS data are in mm for positional errors and deviations and in degree for angular errors and deviations. IQR: interquartile range; RMS: root-mean-square; ρ: Spearman's rank coefficient of correlation. *: Statistically significantly different from zero ($p \leq 0.05$).

References

1. Anderson, K.C.; Buehler, K.C.; Markel, D.C. Computer assisted navigation in total knee arthroplasty: Comparison with conventional methods. *J. Arthroplast.* **2005**, *20*, 132–138. [CrossRef] [PubMed]
2. Choong, P.F.; Dowsey, M.M.; Stoney, J.D. Does accurate anatomical alignment result in better function and quality of life? Comparing conventional and computer-assisted total knee arthroplasty. *J. Arthroplast.* **2009**, *24*, 560–569. [CrossRef] [PubMed]
3. Jacofsky, D.J.; Allen, M. Robotics in Arthroplasty: A Comprehensive Review. *J. Arthroplast.* **2016**, *31*, 2353–2363. [CrossRef] [PubMed]
4. Bautista, M.; Manrique, J.; Hozack, W.J. Robotics in Total Knee Arthroplasty. *J. Knee Surg.* **2019**, *32*, 600–606. [CrossRef]
5. Cosendey, K.; Stanovici, J.; Mahlouly, J.; Omoumi, P.; Jolles, B.M.; Favre, J. Bone Cuts Accuracy of a System for Total Knee Arthroplasty including an Active Robotic Arm. *J. Clin. Med.* **2021**, *10*, 3714. [CrossRef]
6. Stulberg, B.N.; Zadzilka, J.D.; Kreuzer, S.; Kissin, Y.D.; Liebelt, R.; Long, W.J.; Campanelli, V. Safe and effective use of active robotics for TKA: Early results of a multicenter study. *J. Orthop.* **2021**, *26*, 119. [CrossRef]
7. Catani, F.; Biasca, N.; Ensini, A.; Leardini, A.; Bianchi, L.; Digennaro, V.; Giannini, S. Alignment Deviation Between Bone Resection and Final Implant Positioning in Computer-Navigated Total Knee Arthroplasty. *J. Bone Jt. Surg.* **2008**, *90*, 765–771. [CrossRef]
8. Chua, K.H.Z.; Chen, Y.; Lingaraj, K. Navigated total knee arthroplasty: Is it error-free? *Knee Surg. Sports Traumatol. Arthrosc.* **2014**, *22*, 643–649. [CrossRef]
9. Seo, S.S.; Kim, C.W.; Lee, C.R.; Seo, J.H.; Kim, D.H.; Kim, O.G.; Min, Y.K. Does final component alignment correlate with alignment of the bone resection surfaces in cemented total knee arthroplasty? *Knee Surg. Sports Traumatol. Arthrosc.* **2018**, *26*, 1436–1444. [CrossRef] [PubMed]
10. Hampp, E.L.; Chughtai, M.; Scholl, L.Y.; Sodhi, N.; Bhowmik-Stoker, M.; Jacofsky, D.J.; Mont, M.A. Robotic-arm assisted total knee arthroplasty demonstrated greater accuracy and precision to plan compared with manual techniques. *J. Knee Surg.* **2019**, *32*, 239–250. [CrossRef] [PubMed]
11. Koulalis, D.; O'Loughlin, P.F.; Plaskos, C.; Kendoff, D.; Pearle, A.D. Adjustable cutting blocks for computer-navigated total knee arthroplasty: A cadaver study. *J. Arthroplast.* **2010**, *25*, 807–811. [CrossRef]
12. Seidenstein, A.; Birmingham, M.; Foran, J.; Ogden, S. Better accuracy and reproducibility of a new robotically-assisted system for total knee arthroplasty compared to conventional instrumentation: A cadaveric study. *Knee Surg. Sports Traumatol. Arthrosc.* **2021**, *29*, 859–866. [CrossRef]
13. Favre, J.; Babel, H.; Cavinato, A.; Blazek, K.; Jolles, B.M.; Andriacchi, T.P. Analyzing Femorotibial Cartilage Thickness Using Anatomically Standardized Maps: Reproducibility and Reference Data. *J. Clin. Med.* **2021**, *10*, 461. [CrossRef]
14. Große Hokamp, N.; Eck, B.; Siedek, F.; Pinto Dos Santos, D.; Holz, J.A.; Maintz, D.; Haneder, S. Quantification of metal artifacts in computed tomography: Methodological considerations. *Quant. Imaging Med. Surg.* **2020**, *10*, 1033–1044. [CrossRef]
15. Boas, F.E.; Fleischmann, D. CT artifacts: Causes and reduction techniques. *Imaging Med.* **2012**, *4*, 229–240. [CrossRef]
16. Veldpaus, F.E.; Woltring, H.J.; Dortmans, L.J.M.G. A least-squares algorithm for the equiform transformation from spatial marker co-ordinates. *J. Biomech.* **1988**, *21*, 45–54. [CrossRef] [PubMed]
17. Victor, J.; Van Doninck, D.; Labey, L.; Innocenti, B.; Parizel, P.M.; Bellemans, J. How precise can bony landmarks be determined on a CT scan of the knee? *Knee* **2009**, *16*, 358–365. [CrossRef]
18. Sikorski, J.M. Alignment in total knee replacement. *J. Bone Jt. Surg. Br.* **2008**, *90*, 1121–1127. [CrossRef] [PubMed]
19. Jenny, J.-Y.; Clemens, U.; Kohler, S.; Kiefer, H.; Konermann, W.; Miehlke, R.K. Consistency of implantation of a total knee arthroplasty with a non--image-based navigation system: A case-control study of 235 cases compared with 235 conventionally implanted prostheses. *J. Arthroplast.* **2005**, *20*, 832–839. [CrossRef] [PubMed]
20. Laskin, R.S.; Beksaç, B. Computer-assisted navigation in TKA: Where we are and where we are going. *Clin. Orthop. Relat. Res.* **2006**, *452*, 127–131. [CrossRef] [PubMed]
21. Elliott, J.; Shatrov, J.; Fritsch, B.; Parker, D. Robotic-assisted knee arthroplasty: An evolution in progress. A concise review of the available systems and the data supporting them. *Arch. Orthop. Trauma Surg.* **2021**, *141*, 2099–2117. [CrossRef] [PubMed]
22. Mancino, F.; Cacciola, G.; Malahias, M.A.; De Filippis, R.; De Marco, D.; Di Matteo, V.; Gu, A.; Sculco, P.K.; Maccauro, G.; De Martino, I. What are the benefits of robotic-assisted total knee arthroplasty over conventional manual total knee arthroplasty? A systematic review of comparative studies. *Orthop. Rev.* **2020**, *12*, 15–22. [CrossRef]
23. Casper, M.; Mitra, R.; Khare, R.; Jaramaz, B.; Hamlin, B.; McGinley, B.; Mayman, D.; Headrick, J.; Urish, K.; Gittins, M.; et al. Accuracy assessment of a novel image-free handheld robot for Total Knee Arthroplasty in a cadaveric study. *Comput. Assist. Surg.* **2018**, *23*, 14–20. [CrossRef] [PubMed]
24. Parratte, S.; Price, A.J.; Jeys, L.M.; Jackson, W.F.; Clarke, H.D. Accuracy of a new robotically assisted technique for total knee arthroplasty: A cadaveric study. *J. Arthroplast.* **2019**, *34*, 2799–2803. [CrossRef] [PubMed]

Disclaimer/Publisher's Note: The statements, opinions and data contained in all publications are solely those of the individual author(s) and contributor(s) and not of MDPI and/or the editor(s). MDPI and/or the editor(s) disclaim responsibility for any injury to people or property resulting from any ideas, methods, instructions or products referred to in the content.

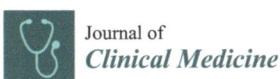

Systematic Review

Greater Risk of Periprosthetic Joint Infection Associated with Prolonged Operative Time in Primary Total Knee Arthroplasty: Meta-Analysis of 427,361 Patients

Kyun-Ho Shin [1,*], Jin-Ho Kim [1] and Seung-Beom Han [2]

1. Department of Orthopedic Surgery, Yeson Hospital, Bucheon 14555, Republic of Korea; jhkayo@naver.com
2. Department of Orthopedic Surgery, Anam Hospital, Korea University College of Medicine, Seoul 02841, Republic of Korea; oahan@korea.ac.kr
* Correspondence: kyunho.shin@gmail.com; Tel.: +82-10-6235-9168

Abstract: Background/Objectives: Periprosthetic joint infection (PJI) is a severe complication in total knee arthroplasty (TKA) with catastrophic outcomes. The relationship between prolonged operative times and PJI remains debated. This meta-analysis investigated the link between prolonged operative times and the risk of PJI in primary TKA. **Methods:** A comprehensive search of the MEDLINE/PubMed, Cochrane Library, and EMBASE databases was conducted to identify studies comparing the incidence of PJI in TKAs with prolonged versus short operative times, as well as those comparing operative times in TKAs with and without PJI. Pooled standardized mean differences (SMD) in operative times between groups with and without PJI or surgical site infections (SSI), including superficial SSIs and PJIs, were analyzed. Additionally, the pooled odds ratios (OR) for PJI in TKAs with operative times exceeding 90 or 120 min were examined. **Results:** Seventeen studies involving 427,361 patients were included. Significant differences in pooled mean operative times between the infected and non-infected TKA groups were observed (PJI, pooled SMD = 0.38, $p < 0.01$; SSI, pooled SMD = 0.72, $p < 0.01$). A higher risk of PJI was noted in surgeries lasting over 90 or 120 min compared to those of shorter duration (90 min, pooled OR = 1.50, $p < 0.01$; 120 min, pooled OR = 1.56, $p < 0.01$). **Conclusions:** An association between prolonged operative time and increased risk of PJI in primary TKA has been established. Strategies for infection prevention should encompass thorough preoperative planning aimed at minimizing factors that contribute to prolonged operative times.

Keywords: total knee arthroplasty; prosthesis-related infections; surgical wound infection; operative time; periprosthetic joint infection

1. Introduction

Periprosthetic joint infection (PJI) stands as one of the most severe complications of primary total knee arthroplasty (TKA), often resulting in catastrophic consequences [1–5]. Established risk factors for PJI include elevated body mass index, diabetes mellitus, urinary tract infections, allogenic blood transfusion, and rheumatoid arthritis [4–8]. However, these factors are largely non-modifiable, particularly in patients with severe arthritis, for whom surgery should not be delayed.

In recent decades, increasing evidence has suggested that operative time is an independent risk factor of surgical site infection (SSI) in various surgical procedures [9]. From a surgeon's point of view, operative time is a potentially modifiable factor, in contrast to patient-related factors. However, in the TKA population, previous studies on operative time as a risk factor of PJI have reported conflicting results. Several studies have demonstrated that longer surgeries are associated with increased risk for infection [10–16], whereas other studies have failed to report such an association [17–22].

To the best of our knowledge, no previous study has conducted a comprehensive review to assess and quantify the association between operative time and PJI in primary

TKA. Given the impact of PJIs on patient outcomes and healthcare burdens, the aim of this meta-analysis was to systematically synthesize the relevant literature that reported on the association between operative time and PJI and quantify the magnitude of the risk of prolonged operative time in patients undergoing primary TKA. We hypothesized that prolonged operative time would be associated with a greater risk of developing PJI following primary TKA. This study underscores the critical importance of managing operative duration in TKA procedures, offering clear guidelines that may help reduce the incidence of PJI, thereby enhancing patient recovery and optimizing resource utilization in clinical settings.

2. Materials and Methods

2.1. Search Strategy

This meta-analysis followed the Preferred Reporting Items for Systematic Reviews and Meta-Analyses (PRISMA) guidelines [23]. This study is registered with the ResearchRegistry, and the unique identifying number is reviewregistry1823.

We performed an electronic literature search of three online databases, namely, Medline/PubMed, the Cochrane Central Register of Controlled Trials, and EMBASE. The last electronic search was performed on 30 July 2023. No restrictions were applied, including the publication language, study period, or sample size. We entered the following Medical Subject Headings (MeSH) terms and key terms in all fields of the search engines: "total knee replacement" OR " total knee arthroplasty" OR "arthroplasty, replacement, knee" [MeSH term] AND "infection" AND "Operative Time" [MeSH term] OR "operative time" OR "operating time" OR "operating times" OR "operating room time" OR "operating room times" OR "surgery time" OR "surgery times" OR "surgical time" OR "surgical times" OR "surgical duration" OR "operation duration" OR "operative duration" OR "surgery duration" or "duration of surgery" or "duration of operation" or "time of operation" or "time of surgery." Following the initial electronic search, the relevant articles and their references were manually searched to identify other suitable articles that were not identified during the database search.

2.2. Eligibility Criteria and Study Selection

We selected studies that were eligible on the basis of the following predefined criteria: (1) studies that reported the outcomes in a cohort of patients who underwent primary TKA and excluded those who underwent revisional TKA; (2) studies that evaluated SSI or PJI and did not include generalized infections such as sepsis, urinary tract infection, or pneumonia; and (3) studies in which the outcomes were based on comparisons of operative times between infected and non-infected patients or on comparisons of infection risks between TKAs with or without prolonged operative times, defined as a cutoff value of 90 min and 120 min, as suggested by the Centers for Disease Control and Prevention to identify post-TKA patients at increased risk of infection [24]. The articles were reviewed by two independent reviewers. During the first stage of screening, the reviewers manually checked the titles and abstracts of all relevant articles. The full texts of the articles were reviewed in the second stage of the screening process to select articles that met the inclusion criteria.

2.3. Data Extraction

Data were extracted according to the following descriptive information provided in the included trials: (1) study characteristics, including the author names, year of publication, study design, level of evidence, and journal title; (2) composition of the study cohort; (3) definition of infection; (4) definition of operative time; (5) controlled variables other than operative times; and (6) follow-up period. In the case of disagreement between the reviewers with respect to the data collected, the extracted data were subsequently cross-checked for accuracy.

2.4. Quality Assessment

Each of the selected studies was evaluated by two independent authors for methodological quality, first independently, and then by consensus. The Newcastle–Ottawa assessment scale was used to assess the methodological quality of the case–control studies [25,26]. The Newcastle–Ottawa assessment scale comprises selection (four categories), comparability, (one category), and outcome domains (three categories). A maximum of one star was assigned for each category within the selection and outcome domains, and a maximum of two stars was given for comparability. Studies with scores ≥ 7 were considered to have a low risk of bias; those with scores 4–6 were considered to have a moderate bias risk; and those with scores 4 were considered to have a high bias risk.

2.5. Definition and Outcomes of Interest

Various definitions of SSI and PJI following TKA are available. The Centers for Disease Control and Prevention (CDC) groups SSIs developed within 90 days of the index procedure into superficial (involvement of skin and subcutaneous tissue of the incision) and deep (involvement of fascial and muscle layers of the incision). Deep SSIs are grouped together as deep SSIs and constitute PJI in the context of hip and knee arthroplasty [24]. Additionally, the Musculoskeletal Infection Society (MSIS) workgroup defined algorithmic criteria for the diagnosis of PJI following TKA [27]. In the clinical practice of arthroplasty, surgical infections are generally divided into superficial SSI or deep SSI as PJI [28]. Reoperation, including debridement and removal or exchange of prostheses, is required for the treatment of PJI, while superficial subcutaneous SSI can be treated with antibiotics and incisional drainage if needed. Therefore, in the present study, PJI was defined as either a deep SSI according to the CDC criteria [24], a PJI diagnosed by the MSIS criteria [27], or a deep infection requiring reoperation after TKA. Furthermore, SSI was defined as all infections around the surgical site, including both superficial SSI and PJI.

Two primary outcomes were evaluated: the operative time in infected versus non-infected TKA cases and the incidence rates of PJI at the latest follow-up, with cohorts divided according to operative time cutoffs of 90 and 120 min.

2.6. Statistical Analysis

All data from the included studies were extracted into an Excel spreadsheet (Version number 1808, Microsoft Corporation, Redmond, WA, USA). Statistical analyses were performed using the packages meta (v4.17-0) in R Studio statistics program (v.1.4.1106) [29]. A p-value < 0.05 was set as the threshold for statistical significance. The operative times were statistically compared between the infected and non-infected groups. The data were standardized for intergroup comparisons of the outcomes because the materials and methods used in the included studies were heterogeneous, such as the definition of operative time. The SMD was defined as the difference in mean outcome divided by the standard deviation of the difference in outcome. The SMD and associated 95% CIs were determined for the operative times. Furthermore, the incidence rates of PJI were compared between a group with prolonged operative times and a control group (patients with short operative times respective to the cutoff value). ORs and 95% CIs were calculated as summary statistics for the incidence rate of PJI.

I^2 statistics were calculated to present the percentage of the total variation attributable to the heterogeneity among the included studies. If there was no heterogeneity ($I^2 \leq 50\%$), the fixed-effects model was used to merge the effect sizes. If there was heterogeneity ($I^2 > 50\%$), the random-effects model was used to merge the effect sizes [30]. A Sensitivity analysis was conducted to determine the influence of an individual study on the overall pooled effects using the leave-one-out analysis. Publication bias was investigated by evaluating the funnel plot asymmetry and by using an Egger test [31,32]. Forest plots were used to graphically present the results of individual studies and the respective pooled estimate of the effect size.

3. Results
3.1. Study Selection and Quality Assessment

Figure 1 shows the process of study identification, inclusion, and exclusion. Electronic searches of the PubMed (Medline), EMBASE, and Cochrane Library databases yielded 274, 462, and 344 studies, respectively. After removing 236 duplicate studies, we obtained 844 studies. Four additional publications were identified through manual searching, among which, 792 were further excluded after reading their abstracts and titles. The full texts of 56 studies were reviewed, and 17 studies were finally included in the meta-analysis after applying the inclusion criteria [10,12,15–17,19–22,32–39]. The main characteristics of the 17 individual studies are summarized in Table 1. Ten studies [10,15–17,21,33,34,37,38,40] showed a low risk of bias. The others [12,19,20,22,35,36,39] did not include a description of the adequacy of patient follow-up and showed a moderate risk of bias (Table 2).

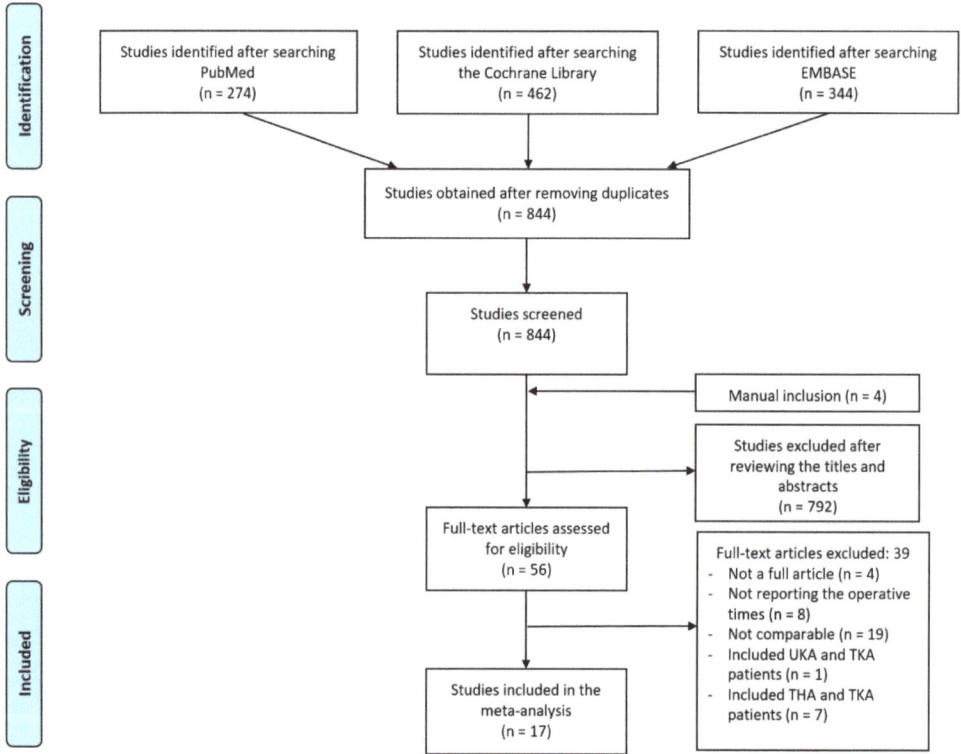

Figure 1. PRISMA flow diagram. PRISMA: Preferred Reporting Items for Systematic Reviews and Meta-Analyses.

Table 1. Baseline characteristics of the included studies.

Author	Publication Year	Study Design	Definition of Infection	Definition of Operative Times	Composition of the Case Group	Number of Patients (Case)	Number of Patients (Control)	Sex (M/F) Case	Sex (M/F) Control	Age (y) Case	Age (y) Control	Duration of Follow-Up	Controlled Confounding Variables	Threshold of Operative Time (min)
Mimema et al. [10] *	2004	Retrospective	CDC criteria	NR	SSI including both superficial and deep infection	22	66	12/10	NR	Median: 68	NR	1 year	Matching for the date of surgery	NR
Namba et al. [12]	2013	Retrospective registry	CDC criteria	NR	Deep surgical site infection	404	55,812	210/194	20,587/35,225	Mean: 66.5	Mean: 67.4	3 months	None	NR
Crowe et al. [22]	2015	Retrospective	CDC criteria	NR	Deep surgical site infection	26	3393	NR	NR	NR	NR	NR	None	114
Lee et al. [33]	2015	Retrospective	Criteria of the Musculoskeletal Infection Society	NR	PJI	8	192	4/4	53/139	Mean: 62.1	NR	2 years	Matching for the year of surgery	NR
Naranje et al. [20]	2015	Retrospective registry	Reoperation for PJI	Time from skin incision to dressing placement	Reoperation for PJI	73	9900	26/47	NR	Mean: 66.2	NR	NR	None	NR
Tayton et al. [34]	2016	Retrospective registry	Reoperation for PJI	NR	Reoperation for PJI	179	64,387	112/67	31,068/33,319	≥65 years (61.5%)	≥65 years (64.7%)	Minimum 1 year	None	90 and 120
Badawy et al. [15]	2017	Retrospective registry	Reoperation for PJI	Time from skin incision to skin closure	Reoperation for PJI	311	27,951	10,186/18,076 (whole cohort)	≥70 years (48.0% of the whole cohort)			Minimum 1 year	None	90
Jung et al. [35]	2017	Retrospective registry	CDC criteria	NR	Deep surgical site infection	44	9437	31/13	4348/5085	≥65 years (52.3%)	≥65 years (68.4%)	3 months	None	90 and 120
George et al. [36]	2018	Retrospective	SSI including superficial and deep infection	Time from skin incision to skin closure	SSI including both superficial and deep infection	1121	139,078	52,855/87,344 (whole cohort)		≥65 years (59.4% of the whole cohort)		1 month	None	NR
Hao et al. [17]	2018	Retrospective	Deep surgical site infection	NR	Deep surgical site infection	16	1145	7/9	221/924	Mean: 62.8	Mean: 64.4	Mean: 1.6 year	None	NR
Teo et al. [37]	2018	Retrospective	Criteria of the Musculoskeletal Infection Society	Time from skin incision to skin closure	SSI including both superficial infection and PJI	10	895	2/8	192/703	Mean: 65.4	Mean: 65.9	2 years	None	NR
Antis et al. [38]	2019	Retrospective	Reoperation for infection	Time from the entry to exit into the operating room	PJI	79	11,761	NR	NR	NR	NR	Mean: 2 years	None	85, 102 and 121
Ravi et al. [16]	2019	Retrospective registry	Reoperation for PJI	NR	Reoperation for PJI	839	91,504	NR	NR	NR	NR	1 year	Age, sex, obesity, primary surgeon, hospital, type of anesthesia	100
Blanco et al. [39]	2020	Retrospective	Criteria of the Musculoskeletal Infection Society	NR	PJI	66	66	20/46	28/38	Mean: 70.1	Mean: 72.4	NR	Matching for the year of surgery	90
Gao et al. [40]	2020	Retrospective	Criteria of the Musculoskeletal Infection Society	NR	PJI	54	108	NR	NR	Mean: 66.8	Mean: 67.2	1 year	Matching for the year of surgery	NR
Iqbal et al. [19]	2020	Retrospective	CDC criteria	NR	PJI	48	4221	28/200	1427/2794	Mean: 61.2	Mean: 61.5	NR	None	NR
Shearer et al. [21]	2020	Retrospective	Criteria of the Musculoskeletal Infection Society	Time from skin incision to skin closure	PJI	31	4114	21/10	2070/2044	Mean: 66.8	Mean: 68.3	1 year	None	NR

M, male; F, female; y, year(s); NR, not reported; CDC, the Centers for Disease Control and Prevention; SSI, surgical site infection, PJI, periprosthetic joint infection. * Reference number.

Table 2. Quality assessment of the included studies.

Author	Publication Year	Selection				Comparability	Outcomes			Overall
		Representativeness of the Exposed Cohort	Selection of the Nonexposed Cohort	Ascertainment of Exposure	Demonstration That the Outcome of Interest Was Not Present at the Start of the Study		Assessment of Outcomes	Sufficient Follow-Up	Adequacy of Follow-Up	
Minnema et al. [10] *	2004	★	★	★	★	★	★	★	★	8
Namba et al. [12]	2013	★	★	★	★	☆	★	☆	★	6
Crowe et al. [22]	2015	★	★	★	★	☆	★	☆	☆	5
Lee et al. [33]	2015	★	★	★	★	★	★	★	★	8
Naranje et al. [20]	2015	★	★	★	★	☆	★	☆	☆	5
Tayton et al. [34]	2016	★	★	★	★	☆	★	★	★	7
Badawy et al. [15]	2017	★	★	★	★	☆	★	★	★	7
Jung et al. [35]	2017	★	★	★	★	☆	★	☆	★	6
George et al. [36]	2018	★	★	★	★	☆	★	★	★	6
Hao et al. [17]	2018	★	★	★	★	☆	★	★	★	7
Teo et al. [37]	2018	★	★	★	★	☆	★	★	★	7
Anis et al. [38]	2019	★	★	★	★	☆	★	★	★	7
Ravi et al. [16]	2019	★	★	★	★	★★	★	★	★	9
Blanco et al. [39]	2020	★	★	★	★	★	★	☆	☆	6
Guo et al. [40]	2020	★	★	★	★	★	★	★	★	8
Iqbal et al. [19]	2020	★	★	★	★	☆	★	☆	☆	5
Shearer et al. [21]	2020	★	★	★	★	☆	★	★	★	7

☆, No star; ★, One star; ★★, Two stars. * Reference number.

3.2. Operative Times in the Primary TKA Cases with and without SSI

Twelve studies comprising 227,547 patients (1905 SSIs) compared the operative times between patients with and without SSI, including both superficial SSI and PJI after TKA [10,12,17,19–21,32,35–39]. The SSI group demonstrated a significantly longer operative time based on our pooled analyses using a random-effects model (pooled standardized mean difference (SMD): 0.38; 95% confidence interval (CI): 0.22–0.53; $p < 0.01$; Figure 2). However, significant heterogeneity was observed ($I^2 = 81\%$; $p < 0.01$).

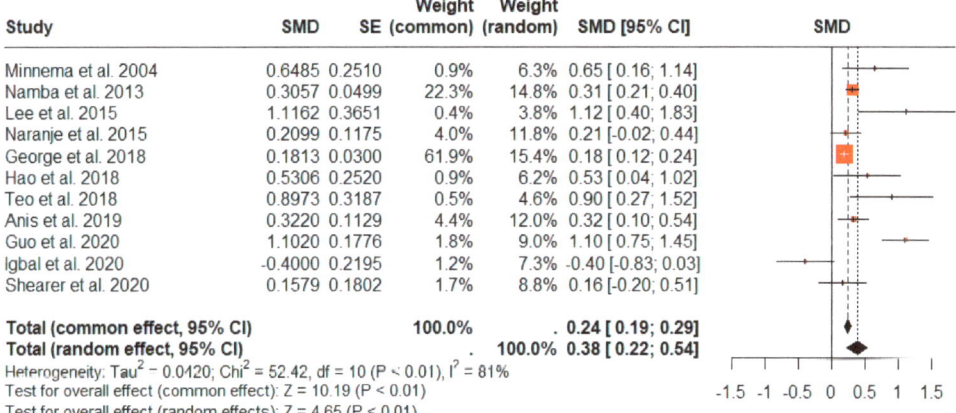

Figure 2. Forest plots showing the operative times of patients with and without surgical site infection. CI, confidence interval; SE, standard error; SMD, standardized mean difference.

3.3. Operative Times in the Primary TKA Cases with and without PJI

Eight studies comprising 85,194 patients (736 PJIs) provided results for the comparison of operative times between patients with and without PJI [12,19–21,32,37–39]. The pooled results demonstrated that a significantly longer operative time was associated with PJI (pooled SMD: 0.72; 95% CI: 0.20–1.24; $p < 0.01$; Figure 3). However, significant heterogeneity was observed ($I^2 = 94\%$; $p < 0.01$).

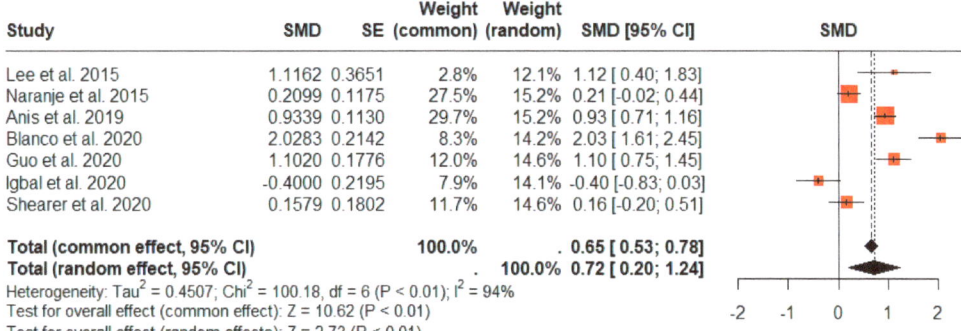

Figure 3. Forest plots showing the operative times of patients with and without periprosthetic joint infection. CI, confidence interval; SE, standard error; SMD, standardized mean difference.

3.4. Comparison of the Incidence of PJI between Operative Times of ≥90 and <90 min

Four studies comprising a total of 194,652 patients compared the incidence rate of PJI in patients divided according to a 90 min cutoff for operative time [15,16,34,35]. The group with longer operative times had a significantly higher prevalence of PJI based on our pooled analysis (pooled odds ratio (OR): 1.50; 95% CI: 1.31–1.73; *p* < 0.01; Figure 4).

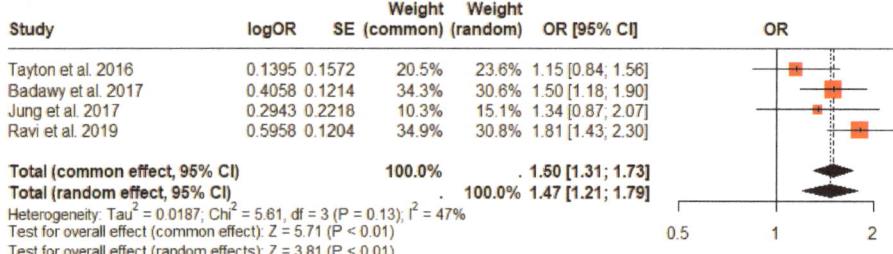

Figure 4. Forest plots comparing the incidence of periprosthetic joint infection in patients with operative times ≥90 min vs. <90 min. CI, confidence interval; OR, odds ratio; SE, Standard error.

3.5. Comparison of the Incidence of PJI between Operative Times of ≥120 and <120 min

Four studies comprising a total of 89,306 patients compared the incidence rate of PJI in patients divided according to a 120 min cutoff for operative time [22,34,35,38]. The group with longer operative times had a significantly higher prevalence of PJI based on our pooled analysis (pooled OR: 1.56; 95% CI: 1.12–2.16; *p* < 0.01; Figure 5).

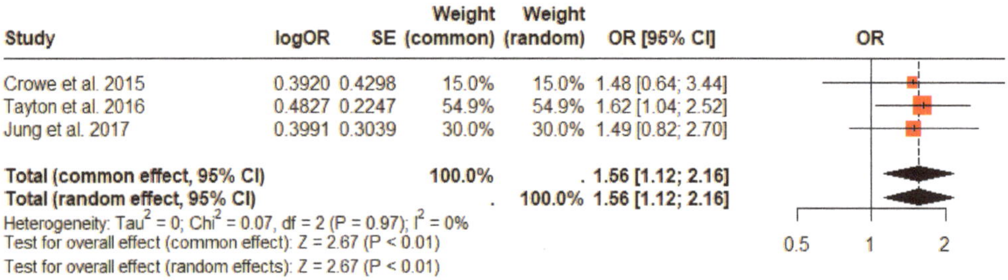

Figure 5. Forest plots comparing the incidence of periprosthetic joint infection between patients with operative times of ≥120 and <120 min. CI, confidence interval; OR, odds ratio; SE, Standard error.

3.6. Sensitivity Analyses and Publication Bias

Sensitivity analysis was conducted on selected studies to evaluate the impact of individual studies on the overall results. The analysis revealed that the data from one study [39] significantly influenced the pooled results for operative times between TKAs with and without SSIs. Another study [12] similarly impacted the pooled results for operative times between TKAs with and without PJIs, as shown in Figures S1 and S2. As a result, these studies were excluded from their respective meta-analyses. Substantial heterogeneity was observed in the pooled risk of PJI associated with the 120 min operative time cutoff. The sensitivity analysis highlighted the study by Anis et al. [38] as a potential source of this heterogeneity. As a result, this study was excluded from the meta-analysis, as detailed in Figure S3. Furthermore, no evidence of publication bias was detected with the Egger regression-based test (all *p*-values > 0.05).

4. Discussion

The present meta-analysis showed that prolonged operative time was associated with a greater risk of PJI in patients undergoing primary TKA. These findings suggest the need for increasing the effort to reduce operative times during TKA. To the best of our knowledge, this is the only published meta-analysis that focuses solely on the incidence of PJI in relation to extended operating times in a primary TKA population.

SSI or PJI after primary TKA requires additional debridement surgery or two-staged revisional arthroplasty, which results in a longer hospital stay, increased morbidity and mortality, and a consequent socioeconomic burden [1–5,7,41]. Efforts to reduce the incidence rates of PJI and SSI after TKA have become increasingly important, and a thorough understanding of modifiable risk factors is essential. Compared with the various patient-related risk factors, such as obesity, diabetes mellitus, and history of operation, operative time is easily assessable and potentially modifiable [4–8].

The exact mechanism by which prolonged operative time increases the incidence rate of infection is multifactorial and poorly understood. With prolonged operative time, open incisions are exposed to microorganisms in the operative environment for a longer period, thus increasing the risk of bacterial contamination [42–45]. Moreover, a longer operative time predisposes patients to an increased risk of tissue desiccation, which may also increase the probability of contamination [46]. Prolonged operative time is also associated with a longer tourniquet time, which can cause persistent wound hypoxia and may increase susceptibility to infection [47,48]. Furthermore, the tissue concentrations of antibiotics decrease as the operative time increases and may be insufficient if the antibiotics are not re-administered during the surgical procedures [49–52].

Many potential factors can affect the operative time, including the complexity of the individual case, experience and fatigue of the surgeon, experience of the operating room staff, implant type, and use of cement. Anis et al. demonstrated that younger age, male sex, higher body mass index, low-volume surgeons, and use of antibiotic cements were significantly associated with longer operative times [38]. Furthermore, relationships between minimally invasive approaches, use of computer navigation, and prolonged operative time have been suggested [20,53,54]. Although none of the factors influencing the increase in operative time can be modified, preoperative planning, procedure efficiency, and surgeon education should be optimized to minimize the impact of operating time on the incidence of PJI where possible [55].

Although identifying a cutoff value for a prolonged operative time is important for surgeons to reduce the risk for PJI, no specific value has been defined due to variation among previous studies. Instead, the pooled risk of prolonged operative time was analyzed in accordance with the National Nosocomial Infections Surveillance guidelines by the Centers for Disease Control and Prevention, which recommends a cutoff value of 120 min as the 75th percentile of operative times [24]. However, with advancement in surgical techniques and instruments, a primary TKA is usually performed in around 90 min in expert hands [16,20,36]. As previous studies recommended a shorter cutoff value for prolonged operative times from 80 to 110 min [15,16,34,35,38,39], the pooled risk of prolonged operative time using the 90 min cutoff was further analyzed. The results support that orthopedic surgeons should consider the risk of PJI in cases with prolonged operative times and should aim to reduce the duration where possible.

The present study has both strengths and limitations. One strength is the comprehensive literature search, which included numerous observational studies. Moreover, the association between operative time and PJI was established through quantitative meta-analyses. However, several limitations should be noted: First, only retrospective studies with a low level of evidence were included, leading to some inherent heterogeneity. Despite this, the large cohort sizes and validated reporting systems in national surveillance or registry databases provide reliable data regarding surgical outcomes. Second, significant differences existed in the definitions of operative time, SSI, and PJI, as well as the follow-up durations across studies. This heterogeneity necessitates cautious interpretation of the results. However, the consistency of PJI risk at the 90 and 120 min operative time cutoffs was maintained across studies through sensitivity analysis. Third, operative time is closely associated with tourniquet time, a potential risk factor for increased PJI in prolonged operative cases [47,48]. While some surgeons perform TKA without tourniquets, making the relationship between tourniquet time and PJI clinically important, this study could not analyze the pooled risk of prolonged tourniquet times. Future large cohort studies with controlled confounding factors are needed to conclude the association between operative and tourniquet times and the risk of PJI. Fourth, antibiotic practices can significantly alter the risk of SSIs and PJIs [56,57]. However, the absence of data on antibiotic redosing and extended antibiotic prophylaxis limited our ability to perform a subanalysis on these factors. Furthermore, longer operative times are often correlated with technical problems during surgery, such as higher BMI, which are independent risk factors for PJI. These factors were not comprehensively controlled for in our analysis, highlighting the need for future research to account for such confounders.

5. Conclusions

In conclusion, the prolonged operative time was significantly associated with the incidence of PJI and SSI after primary TKA. The risk of PJI was also significantly increased in patients with operative times >90 or 120 min compared to those <90 or 120 min, respectively. Identifying a potentially modifiable risk factor such as operative time is important to achieve better patient outcomes. Given the considerable impact of PJIs and SSIs on patient outcomes and the socioeconomic burden, strategies for infection prevention should incorporate preoperative planning and minimize factors that contribute to a prolonged operative time.

Supplementary Materials: The following supporting information can be downloaded at: https://www.mdpi.com/article/10.3390/jcm13113046/s1, Figure S1: Sensitivity analysis for operative times between TKAs with and without SSI; Figure S2: Sensitivity analysis for operative times between TKAs with and without PJI; Figure S3: Sensitivity analysis for the risk of PJI according to a 120-min cutoff for operative time.

Author Contributions: Conceptualization, K.-H.S. and S.-B.H.; formal analysis, K.-H.S. and S.-B.H.; data curation, K.-H.S., J.-H.K. and S.-B.H.; writing—original draft preparation, K.-H.S.; writing—review and editing, K.-H.S. and S.-B.H. All authors have read and agreed to the published version of the manuscript.

Funding: This research received no external funding.

Institutional Review Board Statement: Not applicable.

Informed Consent Statement: Not applicable.

Data Availability Statement: The data presented in this study are available on request from the corresponding author.

Conflicts of Interest: The authors declare no conflicts of interest.

References

1. Lum, Z.C.; Natsuhara, K.M.; Shelton, T.J.; Giordani, M.; Pereira, G.C.; Meehan, J.P. Mortality during total knee periprosthetic joint infection. *J. Arthroplasty* **2018**, *33*, 3783–3788. [CrossRef] [PubMed]
2. Ritter, M.A.; Farris, A. Outcome of infected total joint replacement. *Orthopedics* **2010**, *33*, 149–154. [CrossRef] [PubMed]
3. Barton, C.B.; Wang, D.L.; An, Q.; Brown, T.S.; Callaghan, J.J.; Otero, J.E. Two-stage exchange arthroplasty for periprosthetic joint infection following total hip or knee arthroplasty is associated with high attrition rate and mortality. *J. Arthroplasty* **2020**, *35*, 1384–1389. [CrossRef] [PubMed]
4. Rodríguez-Merchán, E.C.; Liddle, A.D. Epidemiology of the infected total knee arthroplasty: Incidence, causes, and the burden of disease. In *The Infected Total Knee Arthroplasty Prevention, Diagnosis, and Treatment*; Rodríguez-Merchán, E.C., Oussedik, S., Eds.; Springer International Publishing AG: Berlin/Heidelberg, Germany, 2018; pp. 1–10.
5. Rodríguez-Merchán, E.C.; Liddle, A.D. Prevention of periprosthetic joint infection in total knee arthroplasty: Main studies reported between November 2017 and January 2020. *Arch. Bone Jt. Surg.* **2020**, *8*, 465–469. [PubMed]
6. Kim, J.L.; Park, J.H.; Han, S.B.; Cho, I.Y.; Jang, K.M. Allogeneic blood transfusion is a significant risk factor for surgical-site infection following total hip and knee arthroplasty: A meta-analysis. *J. Arthroplast.* **2017**, *32*, 320–325. [CrossRef] [PubMed]
7. Pulido, L.; Ghanem, E.; Joshi, A.; Purtill, J.J.; Parvizi, J. Periprosthetic joint infection: The incidence, timing, and predisposing factors. *Clin. Orthop. Relat. Res.* **2008**, *466*, 1710–1715. [CrossRef] [PubMed]
8. Lenguerrand, E.; Whitehouse, M.R.; Beswick, A.D.; Kunutsor, S.K.; Foguet, P.; Porter, M.; Blom, A.W. Risk factors associated with revision for prosthetic joint infection following knee replacement: An observational cohort study from England and Wales. *Lancet Infect. Dis.* **2019**, *19*, 589–600. [CrossRef]

9. Cheng, H.; Chen, B.P.; Soleas, I.M.; Ferko, N.C.; Cameron, C.G.; Hinoju, P. Prolonged operative duration increases risk of surgical site infections: A systematic review. *Surg. Infect.* **2017**, *18*, 722–735. [CrossRef]
10. Minnema, B.; Vearncombe, M.; Augustin, A.; Gollish, J.; Simor, A.E. Risk factors for surgical-site infection following primary total knee arthroplasty. *Infect. Control Hosp. Epidemio* **2004**, *25*, 477–480. [CrossRef]
11. Mraovic, B.; Suh, D.; Jacovides, C.; Parvizi, J. Perioperative hyperglycemia and postoperative infection after lower limb arthroplasty. *J. Diabetes Sci. Technol.* **2011**, *5*, 412–418. [CrossRef]
12. Namba, R.S.; Inacio, M.C.; Paxton, E.W. Risk factors associated with deep surgical site infections after primary total knee arthroplasty: An analysis of 56,216 knees. *J. Bone Jt. Surg. Am.* **2013**, *95*, 775–782. [CrossRef] [PubMed]
13. Peersman, G.; Laskin, R.; Davis, J.; Peterson, M.G.; Richart, T. Prolonged operative time correlates with increased infection rate after total knee arthroplasty. *HSS J.* **2006**, *2*, 70–72. [CrossRef] [PubMed]
14. Song, K.H.; Kim, E.S.; Kim, Y.K.; Jin, H.Y.; Jeong, S.Y.; Kwak, Y.G.; Cho, Y.K.; Sung, J.; Lee, Y.S.; Oh, H.B.; et al. Differences in the risk factors for surgical site infection between total hip arthroplasty and total knee arthroplasty in the Korean Nosocomial Infections Surveillance System (KONIS). *Infect. Control Hosp. Epidemiol.* **2012**, *33*, 1086–1093. [CrossRef] [PubMed]
15. Badawy, M.; Espehaug, B.; Fenstad, A.M.; Indrekvam, K.; Dale, H.; Havelin, L.I.; Furnes, O. Patient and surgical factors affecting procedure duration and revision risk due to deep infection in primary total knee arthroplasty. *BMC Musculoskelet. Disord.* **2017**, *18*, 544. [CrossRef] [PubMed]
16. Ravi, B.; Jenkinson, R.; O'Heireamhoin, S.; Austin, P.C.; Aktar, S.; Leroux, T.S.; Paterson, M.; Redelmeier, D.A. Surgical duration is associated with an increased risk of periprosthetic infection following total knee arthroplasty: A population-based retrospective cohort study. *eClinicalMedicine* **2019**, *16*, 74–80. [CrossRef] [PubMed]
17. Hao, L.; Zhang, Y.; Song, W.; Ma, T.; Wang, J.; Cheng, H.; Li, K.; Qin, S. Risk factors for infection following primary total knee replacement. *Biomed. Res.* **2018**, *29*, 715–723. [CrossRef]
18. Hijas-Gómez, A.I.; Lucas, W.C.; Checa-García, A.; Martínez-Martín, J.; Fahandezh-Saddi, H.; Gil-de-Miguel, Á.; Durán-Poveda, M.; Rodríguez-Caravaca, G. Surgical site infection incidence and risk factors in knee arthroplasty: A 9-year prospective cohort study at a university teaching hospital in Spain. *Am. J. Infect. Control* **2018**, *46*, 1335–1340. [CrossRef] [PubMed]
19. Iqbal, F.; Shafiq, B.; Zamir, M.; Noor, S.; Memon, N.; Memon, N.; Dina, T.K. Micro-organisms and risk factors associated with prosthetic joint infection following primary total knee replacement-our experience in Pakistan. *Int. Orthop.* **2020**, *44*, 283–289. [CrossRef] [PubMed]
20. Naranje, S.; Lendway, L.; Mehle, S.; Gioe, T.J. Does operative time affect infection rate in primary total knee arthroplasty? *Clin. Orthop. Relat. Res.* **2015**, *473*, 64–69. [CrossRef]
21. Shearer, J.; Agius, L.; Burke, N.; Rahardja, R.; Young, S.W. BMI is a Better Predictor of Periprosthetic Joint Infection Risk Than Local Measures of Adipose Tissue After TKA. *J. Arthroplasty* **2020**, *35*, S313–S318. [CrossRef]
22. Crowe, B.; Payne, A.; Evangelista, P.J.; Stachel, A.; Phillips, M.S.; Slover, J.D.; Inneh, I.A.; Iorio, R.; Bosco, J.A. Risk Factors for Infection Following Total Knee Arthroplasty: A Series of 3836 Cases from One Institution. *J. Arthroplasty* **2015**, *30*, 2275–2278. [CrossRef] [PubMed]
23. Moher, D.; Liberati, A.; Tetzlaff, J.; Altman, D.G.; PRISMA Group. Preferred reporting items for systematic reviews and meta-analyses: The PRISMA statement. *PLoS Med.* **2009**, *6*, e1000097. [CrossRef] [PubMed]
24. Centers for Disease Control and Prevention-National Healthcare Safety Networks (CDC/NHSN). Procedure-Associated Module—Surgical Site Infection (SSI) Event. 2015. Available online: http://www.cdc.gov/nhsn/pdfs/pscmanual/9pscssicurrent.pdf (accessed on 1 August 2023).
25. Stang, A. Critical evaluation of the Newcastle-Ottawa scale for the assessment of the quality of nonrandomized studies in meta-analyses. *Eur. J. Epidemiol.* **2011**, *25*, 603–605. [CrossRef] [PubMed]
26. Wells, G.A.; SHEA, B.; O'connell, D.; Peterson, J.; Welch, V.; Losos, M.; Tugwell, P. The Newcastle-Ottawa Scale (NOS) for Assessing the Quality of Nonrandomized Studies in Meta-Analyses. Available online: http://www.ohri.ca/programs/clinical_epidemiology/oxford.htm (accessed on 30 July 2023).
27. Parvizi, J.; Zmistowski, B.; Berbari, E.F.; Bauer, T.W.; Springer, B.D.; Della Valle, C.J.; Garvin, K.L.; Mont, M.A.; Wongworawat, M.D.; Zalavras, C.G. New definition for periprosthetic joint infection: From the Workgroup of the Musculoskeletal Infection Society. *Clin. Orthop. Relat. Res.* **2011**, *469*, 2992–2994. [CrossRef] [PubMed]
28. Amanatullah, D.; Dennis, D.; Oltra, E.G.; Gomes, L.S.M.; Goodman, S.B.; Hamlin, B.; Hansen, E.; Hashemi-Nejad, A.; Holst, D.C.; Komnos, G.; et al. Hip and Knee Section, Diagnosis, Definitions: Proceedings of International Consensus on Orthopedic Infections. *J. Arthroplasty* **2019**, *34*, S329–S337. [CrossRef] [PubMed]
29. RStudio Team. RStudio: Integrated Development for R. RStudio, PBC: Boston, MA, USA, 2020. Available online: http://www.rstudio.com/ (accessed on 30 July 2023).
30. DerSimonian, R.; Laird, N. Meta-analysis in clinical trials. *Control Clin. Trials* **1986**, *7*, 177–188. [CrossRef] [PubMed]
31. Egger, M.; Smith, G.D.; Schneider, M.; Minder, C. Bias in meta-analysis detected by a simple, graphical test. *BMJ* **1997**, *315*, 629–634. [CrossRef] [PubMed]
32. Duval, S.; Tweedie, R. Trim and fill: A simple funnel-plot-based method of testing and adjusting for publication bias in meta-analysis. *Biometrics* **2000**, *56*, 455–463. [CrossRef] [PubMed]
33. Lee, Q.J.; Mak, W.P.; Wong, Y.C. Risk factors for periprosthetic joint infection in total knee arthroplasty. *J. Orthop. Surg.* **2015**, *23*, 282–286. [CrossRef]

34. Tayton, E.R.; Frampton, C.; Hooper, G.J.; Young, S.W. The impact of patient and surgical factors on the rate of infection after primary total knee arthroplasty: An analysis of 64,566 joints from the New Zealand Joint Registry. *Bone Jt. J.* **2016**, *98-B*, 334–340. [CrossRef]
35. Jung, P.; Morris, A.J.; Zhu, M.; Roberts, S.A.; Frampton, C.; Young, S.W. BMI is a key risk factor for early periprosthetic joint infection following total hip and knee arthroplasty. *N. Z. Med. J.* **2017**, *130*, 24–34. [PubMed]
36. George, J.; Mahmood, B.; Sultan, A.A.; Sodhi, N.; Mont, M.A.; Higuera, C.A.; Stearns, K.L. How Fast Should a Total Knee Arthroplasty Be Performed? An Analysis of 140,199 Surgeries. *J. Arthroplasty* **2018**, *33*, 2616–2622. [CrossRef] [PubMed]
37. Teo, B.J.X.; Yeo, W.; Chong, H.C.; Tan, A.H.C. Surgical site infection after primary total knee arthroplasty is associated with a longer duration of surgery. *J. Orthop. Surg.* **2018**, *26*, 2309499018785647. [CrossRef]
38. Anis, H.K.; Sodhi, N.; Klika, A.K.; Mont, M.A.; Barsoum, W.K.; Higuera, C.A.; Molloy, R.M. Is Operative Time a Predictor for Post-Operative Infection in Primary Total Knee Arthroplasty? *J. Arthroplasty* **2019**, *34*, S331–S336. [CrossRef] [PubMed]
39. Blanco, J.F.; Díaz, A.; Melchor, F.R.; da Casa, C.; Pescador, D. Risk factors for periprosthetic joint infection after total knee arthroplasty. *Arch. Orthop. Trauma. Surg.* **2020**, *140*, 239–245. [CrossRef] [PubMed]
40. Guo, H.; Xu, C.; Chen, J. Risk factors for periprosthetic joint infection after primary artificial hip and knee joint replacements. *J. Infect. Dev. Ctries.* **2020**, *14*, 565–571. [CrossRef]
41. Zmistowski, B.; Karam, J.A.; Durinka, J.B.; Casper, D.S.; Parvizi, J. Periprosthetic joint infection increases the risk of one-year mortality. *J. Bone Jt. Surg. Am.* **2013**, *95*, 2177–2184. [CrossRef]
42. Whyte, W.; Hodgson, R.; Tinkler, J. The importance of airborne bacterial contamination of wounds. *J. Hosp. Infect.* **1982**, *3*, 123–135. [CrossRef] [PubMed]
43. Lidwell, O.M.; Lowbury, E.J.; Whyte, W.; Blowers, R.; Stanley, S.J.; Lowe, D. Airborne contamination of wounds in joint replacement operations: The relationship to sepsis rates. *J. Hosp. Infect.* **1983**, *4*, 111–131. [CrossRef]
44. Howorth, F.H. Prevention of airborne infection during surgery. *Lancet* **1985**, *1*, 386–388. [CrossRef]
45. Garibaldi, R.A.; Cushing, D.; Lerer, T. Risk factors for postoperative infection. *Am. J. Med.* **1991**, *91*, 158S–163S. [CrossRef] [PubMed]
46. Haridas, M.; Malangoni, M.A. Predictive factors for surgical site infection in general surgery. *Surgery* **2008**, *144*, 496–503. [CrossRef] [PubMed]
47. Abdel-Salam, A.; Eyres, K.S. Effects of tourniquet during total knee arthroplasty. A prospective randomised study. *J. Bone Jt. Surg. Br.* **1995**, *77*, 250–253. [CrossRef] [PubMed]
48. Clarke, M.T.; Longstaff, L.; Edwards, D.; Rushton, N. Tourniquet-induced wound hypoxia after total knee replacement. *J. Bone Jt. Surg. Br.* **2001**, *83*, 40–44. [CrossRef] [PubMed]
49. Alavi, K.; Sturrock, P.R.; Sweeney, W.B.; Maykel, J.A.; Cervera-Servin, J.A.; Tseng, J.; Cook, E.F. A simple risk score for predicting surgical site infections in inflammatory bowel disease. *Dis. Colon. Rectum* **2010**, *53*, 1480–1486. [CrossRef] [PubMed]
50. Malone, D.L.; Genuit, T.; Tracy, J.K.; Gannon, C.; Napolitano, L.M. Surgical site infections: Reanalysis of risk factors. *J. Surg. Res.* **2002**, *103*, 89–95. [CrossRef]
51. Sergeant, G.; Buffet, W.; Fieuws, S.; de Gheldere, C.; Vanclooster, P. Incisional surgical site infections after colorectal surgery: Time to appraise its true incidence. *Acta Chir. Belg.* **2008**, *108*, 513–517. [CrossRef]
52. Tweed, C. Prevention of surgical wound infection: Prophylactic antibiotics in colorectal surgery. *J. Wound Care* **2005**, *14*, 202–205. [CrossRef]
53. King, J.; Stamper, D.L.; Schaad, D.C.; Leopold, S.S. Minimally invasive total knee arthroplasty compared with traditional total knee arthroplasty. Assessment of the learning curve and the postoperative recuperative period. *J. Bone Jt. Surg. Am.* **2007**, *89*, 1497–1503.
54. Lau, R.L.; Perruccio, A.V.; Gandhi, R.; Mahomed, N.N. The role of surgeon volume on patient outcome in total knee arthroplasty: A systematic review of the literature. *BMC Musculoskelet. Disord.* **2012**, *13*, 250. [CrossRef]
55. Maoz, G.; Phillips, M.; Bosco, J.; Slover, J.; Stachel, A.; Inneh, I.; Iorio, R. The Otto Aufranc Award: Modifiable versus nonmodifiable risk factors for infection after hip arthroplasty. *Clin. Orthop. Relat. Res.* **2015**, *473*, 453–459. [CrossRef] [PubMed]
56. Kheir, M.M.; Dilley, J.E.; Ziemba-Davis, M.; Meneghini, R.M. The AAHKS Clinical Research Award: Extended Oral Antibiotics Prevent Periprosthetic Joint Infection in High-Risk Cases: 3855 Patients With 1-Year Follow-Up. *J. Arthroplasty* **2021**, *36*, S18–S25. [CrossRef] [PubMed]
57. Dasari, S.P.; Kanumuri, S.D.; Yang, J.; Manner, P.A.; Fernando, N.D.; Hernandez, N.M. Extended Prophylactic Antibiotics for Primary and Aseptic Revision Total Joint Arthroplasty: A Meta-Analysis. *J. Arthroplasty.* **2024**, *17*, S0883-5403(24)00014-7. [CrossRef] [PubMed]

Disclaimer/Publisher's Note: The statements, opinions and data contained in all publications are solely those of the individual author(s) and contributor(s) and not of MDPI and/or the editor(s). MDPI and/or the editor(s) disclaim responsibility for any injury to people or property resulting from any ideas, methods, instructions or products referred to in the content.

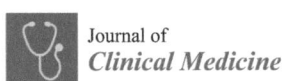

Article

Multivariate Analysis of Risk Factors for In-Hospital Dislocation Following Primary Total Hip Arthroplasty

Hunter B. Jones [1,*], Andrew J. Hinkle [1], Yida Liu [1] and Senthil N. Sambandam [1,2]

[1] Department of Orthopedic Surgery, University of Texas Southwestern Medical Center, 5323 Harry Hines Blvd, Dallas, TX 75390, USA; andrew.hinkle@utsouthwestern.edu (A.J.H.); yida.liu@utsouthwestern.edu (Y.L.); senthil.sambandam@utsouthwestern.edu (S.N.S.)
[2] Department of Orthopedic Surgery, VA North Texas Health Care System, Dallas, TX 75216, USA
* Correspondence: hunter.jones@utsouthwestern.edu

Abstract: Background: Early dislocation following primary total hip arthroplasty (THA) is a rare but devastating complication and represents a source of patient morbidity and financial burden to the healthcare system. The objective of this study was to identify patient characteristics and comorbidities that are associated with increased early in-hospital dislocation rates following primary THA. **Methods:** A retrospective cohort study was conducted using patient data from the Nationwide Inpatient Sample (NIS) database; we identified patients who had undergone THA from 2016 to 2019 and compared those with an early periprosthetic dislocation prior to discharge to those without. The patient characteristics and comorbidities were compared using univariate analysis with a subsequent investigation of statistically significant variables using multivariate analysis. The variables were compared using chi square, Fisher's exact test, and independent sample t-tests with data assessed using odds ratio with 95% confidence intervals. **Results:** A total of 5151 patients sustained an early dislocation compared to 362,743 who did not. Those who sustained an in-hospital dislocation were more likely to share the following characteristics: female sex (OR 1.21, $p < 0.01$), age > 70 (OR 1.45, $p < 0.01$), Caucasian ethnicity (OR 1.22, $p < 0.01$), SLE (OR 1.87, $p < 0.01$), and Parkinson's disease (OR 1.93, $p < 0.01$). Certain characteristics were also associated with decreased odds of having an in-hospital dislocation including elective surgery (OR 0.14, $p < 0.01$), tobacco use (OR 0.8, $p < 0.01$), diabetes without complications (OR 0.87, $p < 0.01$), and a history of heart valve replacement (OR 0.81, $p < 0.01$). The length of stay was significantly longer (4.7 days vs. 2.3 days) as was the total hospital charges (USD $101,517 vs. USD $66,388) for the early in-hospital dislocation group. **Conclusions:** Several patient characteristics and comorbidities are associated with early in-hospital dislocation episodes following total hip arthroplasty including female sex, age > 70, non-elective surgery, SLE, and Parkinson's. This information may be useful to help guide intraoperative implant selection and/or postoperative protocol in select patient populations to limit early instability as well as decrease the financial burden associated with this postoperative complication.

Keywords: total hip arthroplasty; periprosthetic dislocation; hip instability

1. Introduction

Total hip arthroplasty (THA) is a highly effective surgery for patients with degenerative hip joints or femoral neck fractures. Furthermore, it has an excellent track record, leading some to refer to it as the operation of the twentieth century [1]. It has been shown that the annual volume of THAs has increased by close to 177% over the past 20 years. Future projections estimate that 700,000 of these procedures will be performed by the year 2040 in the United States alone [2].

While it was previously understood that aseptic loosening was the most common reason for revision THA (rTHA) [3], recent data suggest that instability has become a more common indication, ranging from 17 to 22% of all revisions [4,5]. Most of these dislocations occur early, within 6 months. Some of the literature suggests that instability within the first two years is responsible for nearly three times as many rTHA procedures as compared to after two years [6].

THA instability is caused by multiple factors that generally relate to patient characteristics, surgical details, and/or postoperative management. Classically, age has been one of the more important patient-related factors, with an increased risk of dislocation at ages over 80 [7,8]. While female sex was previously thought to be a risk factor, the more recent literature suggests this is not the case [9]. Instability is also influenced by the presence of nervous system disorders such as Parkinson's disease [10]. Although different surgical approaches have been considered to result in varying dislocation rates [11], this is generally less agreed upon in the current literature. Surgeon experience along with prosthesis selection/design are two other surgery-related factors that play a role. Lastly, postoperative management is also important for guiding patients in the recovery period after THA. Modalities such as high-risk-position avoidance, assistive devices, and hip abduction orthoses are all important to consider.

The average length of stay following THA reported in database studies is around 2.97 days [12], and there is a small but important subset of patients who sustain in-hospital dislocation in the immediate postoperative period. However, there are very little data examining the incidence during this time period along with the associated financial burden that it imposes on the medical system.

The objective of this study was to identify patient characteristics and comorbidities that are associated with early in-hospital dislocation rates following primary THA.

2. Methods

We utilized a retrospective analysis of the Nationwide Inpatient Sample (NIS) database. We then queried for all patients who underwent primary THA from 2016 to 2019 using International Classification of Disease, Tenth Revision (ICD-10) codes (Table A1). We further stratified this population into two cohorts based on the presence or absence of an in-hospital dislocation following THA. The NIS strictly contains inpatient information only; therefore, data were included from index procedure admission to discharge. Patient demographics such as age, sex, and race were obtained along with length of stay, total charges, and disposition at discharge (routine, short-term hospital stay, alternate facility, death, etc). Select medical comorbidities were also obtained. This study was exempt from IRB approval since the data are publicly available and lack identifying information. To further protect against patient confidentiality, patient values between 1 and 10 were not reported per the healthcare cost and utilization project data agreement.

We used SPSS software version 27.0 (IBM, Armonk, NY, USA) for our statistical analysis. Continuous variables were described using mean value and analyzed with the two-sided independent sample t-test. Categorical variables were described using frequency and analyzed using the chi-square test, although the Fisher's exact test was used for values less than five. Additionally, we utilized multivariate analysis (MVA) for variables that came to show statistically significant associations on univariate analysis (UVA). We calculated the odds ratio (OR) and 95% confidence intervals to assess our variables. We used a p value of 0.05 to define significance.

3. Results

The NIS database identified 367,894 patients who underwent primary THA between 2016 to 2019. Of these, 5151 patients (1.4%) were reported to have sustained an in-hospital dislocation during the same admission.

The average age of those with a dislocation was 68.2 years versus 65.8 years for those without dislocation. Patients in our dislocation cohort had a higher incidence of age over 70 (47.5% vs. 38.4%) (OR 1.45, $p < 0.01$). Patients with a dislocation were more likely to be female (63.2% versus 55.8%) (OR 1.36, $p < 0.01$). Caucasians made up 87.7% of the dislocation group compared to 85.5% of the non-dislocation group (OR 1.2, 95% CI 1.09 to

1.38, $p < 0.01$) while African Americans made up 6.1% of the dislocation group compared to 7.8% of the non-dislocation group (OR 0.76, $p < 0.01$). There was not a significant difference between the remainder of the different ethnicities (Table 1).

Table 1. Patient demographics.

	Dislocation Group	Non-Dislocation Group	OR (95% CI)	p
Average age at admission	68.2 years	65.8 years		
Age > 70	2445 (47.5%)	139,112 (38.4%)	1.45 (1.37, 153)	<0.001
Female sex	3257 (63.2%)	202,485 (55.8%)	1.36 (1.29, 1.44)	<0.001
Ethnicity				
Caucasian	4360 (87.7%)	298,742 (85.5%)	1.21 (1.11, 1.32)	<0.001
African American	301 (6.1%)	27,261 (7.8%)	0.76 (0.68, 0.86)	<0.001
Hispanic	158 3.2%	12,876 (3.7%)	0.86 (0.73, 1.01)	0.06
Asian	48 (1.0%)	3362 (1.0%)	1.01 (0.76, 1.34)	0.97
Native American	21 (0.4%)	1101 (0.3%)	1.34 (0.87, 2.07)	0.18
Other	82 (1.7%)	5941 (1.7%)	1.0	0.99

Only 60.3% of the dislocation group underwent THA as an elective procedure with the rest being non-elective for trauma or other medical indications. This is in comparison to the non-dislocation group with 91.8% being elective procedures (OR 0.14, $p < 0.01$). Patients in the dislocation group were at a significant risk of non-home discharge (Table 2). Furthermore, 0.45% of patients in the dislocation group died during admission compared to 0.09% of the non-dislocation group (OR 5.7, $p < 0.01$). The average length of stay for those with a dislocation was 4.7 days compared to 2.3 days, while the average total hospital charges were USD 101,517 compared to USD 66,388, respectively (Table 2).

Table 2. Admission and disposition characteristics.

	Dislocation Group	Non-Dislocation Group	OR (95% CI)	p
Elective surgery	3099 (60.3%)	332,454 (91.8%)	0.14 (0.13, 0.14)	<0.001
Disposition of patient				
Routine discharge	1296 (25.2%)	141,942 (39.1%)		
Short-term hospital stay	44 (0.9%)	826 (0.23%)		
Intermediate care facility	2137 (41.5%)	65,361 (18.0%)		<0.001
Another type of facility	1636 (31.8%)	153,928 (42.5%)		
Home healthcare	12 (0.2%)	241 (0.07%)		
Against medical advice	23 (0.5%)	309 (0.1%)		
Death during admission	23 (0.5%)	309 (0.1%)	5.26 (3.44, 8.05)	<0.001
Average length of stay	4.7 days	2.3 days		
Average total charges	USD 101,517.00	USD 66,388.00		

Univariate analysis showed that patients in the dislocation group had an increased incidence of CKD (7.6% vs. 5.9%, $p < 0.01$), requirement of dialysis (0.2% vs. 0.1%, $p < 0.01$), systemic lupus erythematosus (SLE) (0.9% vs. 0.5%, $p < 0.01$), Parkinson's disease (1.7% vs. 0.5%, $p < 0.01$), cirrhosis (0.5% vs. 0.3%, $p < 0.01$), history of organ transplant (0.4% vs. 0.2%, $p = 0.01$), presence of pacemaker (2.4% vs. 1.5%, $p < 0.01$), and presence of colostomy (0.2% vs. 0.1%, $p = 0.02$). These patients were also shown to have a decreased incidence of tobacco use (12.2% vs. 17.4%, $p < 0.01$), obesity (19.3% vs. 21.8%, $p < 0.01$), and diabetes (DM) without complications (8.6% vs. 10.0%) (Table 3).

Table 3. Patient comorbidities.

	Dislocation Group	Non-Dislocation Group	OR (95% CI)	p
Tobacco use	629 (12.2%)	63,079 (17.4%)	0.66 (0.61, 0.72)	**<0.001**
Obesity (BMI 30–40)	993 (19.3%)	78,926 (21.8%)	0.86 (0.80, 0.92)	**<0.001**
Morbid obesity (BMI 40–50)	403 (7.8%)	27,675 (7.6%)	1.03 (0.93, 1.14)	0.6
Super obesity (BMI >50)	31 (0.6%)	1615 (0.5%)	1.35 (0.95, 1.93)	0.09
DM w/o complications	441 (8.6%)	36,387 (10.0%)	0.84 (0.76, 0.93)	**<0.001**
DM w/complications	* (0.2%)	704 (0.2%)	0.90 (0.47, 1.74)	0.75
CKD	391 (7.6%)	21,235 (5.9%)	1.32 (1.19, 1.47)	**<0.001**
Dialysis	12 (0.2%)	371 (0.1%)	2.28 (1.28, 4.06)	**0.004**
HIV	* (0.1%)	497 (0.1%)	0.88 (0.53, 1.43)	0.98
Sickle cell disease	* (0.2%)	646 (0.2%)	0.98 (0.51, 1.90)	1
SLE	44 (0.9%)	1640 (0.5%)	1.9 (1.40, 2.56)	**<0.001**
Parkinson's disease	89 (1.7%)	1838 (0.5%)	3.45 (2.79, 4.28)	**<0.001**
Ankylosing spondylitis	* (0.1%)	495 (0.1%)	0.85 (0.38, 1.9)	0.85
Cirrhosis	28 (0.5%)	1106 (0.3%)	1.79 (1.23, 2.60)	**0.002**
Hx of transplant	20 (0.4%)	793 (0.2%)	1.78 (1.14, 2.78)	**0.016**
Hx of CABG	143 (2.8%)	8948 (2.5%)	1.13 (0.96, 1.34)	0.16
Hx of PCI	202 (3.9%)	13,062 (3.6%)	1.09 (0.95, 1.26)	0.22
Hx of heart valve replacement	31 (0.6%)	3090 (0.9%)	0.71 (0.49, 1.01)	0.06
Presence of pacemaker	121 (2.4%)	5436 (1.5%)	1.58 (1.32, 1.90)	**<0.001**
Presence of colostomy	12 (0.2%)	433 (0.1%)	1.95 (1.10, 3.47)	**0.02**
Legally blind	* (0.1%)	315 (0.1%)	1.57 (0.74, 3.31)	0.24
Down syndrome	* (0.0%)	128 (0.0%)	0.55 (0.08, 3.94)	0.46

* Numbers between 1 and 10 were not reported per the healthcare cost and utilization project data agreement.

After multivariate analysis, we found that those who sustained an in-hospital dislocation were more likely to share the following characteristics: female sex (OR 1.21, $p < 0.01$), Caucasian ethnicity (OR 1.22, $p < 0.01$), SLE (OR 1.87, $p < 0.01$), and Parkinson's disease (OR 1.93, $p < 0.01$). Certain characteristics were also associated with decreased odds of having an in-hospital dislocation including elective surgery (OR 0.14, $p < 0.01$), tobacco use (OR 0.8, $p < 0.01$), diabetes without complications (OR 0.87, $p < 0.01$), and history of heart valve replacement (OR 0.81, $p < 0.01$) (Tables 3 and 4).

Table 4. Multivariate analysis.

	OR (95% CI)	p
Female sex	1.21 (1.14, 1.28)	**<0.001**
Caucasian	1.22 (1.09, 1.38)	**<0.001**
African American	0.97 (0.83, 1.14)	0.71
Elective surgery	0.14 (0.14, 0.15)	**<0.001**
Tobacco use	0.80 (0.73, 0.87)	**<0.001**
DM w/o complications	0.87 (0.79, 0.96)	**0.008**
CKD	1.05 (0.94, 1.18)	0.37
Dialysis	1.45 (0.80, 2.63)	0.23
SLE	1.87 (1.37, 2.54)	**<0.001**
Parkinson's disease	1.93 (1.54, 2.43)	**<0.001**
Cirrhosis	1.28 (0.87, 1.88)	0.21
Hx of transplant	1.52 (0.95, 2.41)	0.08
Hx of heart valve replacement	0.57 (0.40, 0.81)	**0.002**
Presence of pacemaker	1.19 (0.98, 1.44)	0.08
Presence of colostomy	1.48 (0.82, 2.65)	0.19

4. Discussion

Our incidence of 1.4% of patients who sustained an in-hospital dislocation following THA was unexpectedly high. A multivariate analysis assessing the risk of dislocation in a Charnley hip replacement by Berry et al. reported a 1% risk at 1 month postoperatively with an approximate 1% increase in risk per year thereafter [13]. In another database study by Gausden et al., it was shown that 1.4% of THA patients had a readmission within 6 months relating to instability [14]. However, their rate is slightly lower than another Medicare database study by Goel et al., who reported a rate of 2.14% [15]. An international study out of the Danish Hip Arthroplasty Registry by Hermansen et al. showed a two-year cumulative incidence of dislocation to range from 2.2% to 4.3%; however, there was significant hospital variation depending on volume [16]. Nevertheless, our incidence of 1.4% of in-hospital dislocation further emphasizes the significance of this issue. No studies specifically looked at rates of dislocation in the immediate postoperative period while still admitted.

Our study was able to highlight several factors that appear to increase the odds of sustaining an early dislocation in the immediate postoperative period, notably older age, female sex, non-elective surgery, SLE, and Parkinson's disease. This is the first study to our knowledge that has evaluated these risk factors specifically in the immediate postoperative period.

Older age has previously been understood to be a risk factor for instability following THA [17,18]. We found an OR of 1.45 in patients over the age of 70. This is in agreement with Berry et al., who noted a relative risk of 1.3 for dislocation in patients over the age of 70 [13]. Some older studies have cited dislocation rates upwards of two to three times higher in patients over the age of 80 [7,8]. However, Gausden et al. did not find a correlation between age and an increased risk for dislocation [14]. Our results would suggest that this is not the case, particularly in the setting of an early in-hospital dislocation with the etiology speculated to be related to poorer tissue quality and a decreased muscular envelope.

The literature regarding female sex as a risk factor has been less agreed upon. Females had previously been reported to be at increased risk of dislocation compared to males, with some studies citing ratios of up to 3:1 [13,19]. However, other studies disagree with this assertion [20]. Our study cites an OR of 1.21, which is in agreement with the majority of the literature on the matter, furthering the hypothesis that there may be a difference in soft tissue laxity and/or postoperative range of motion as the root cause [14].

THA for displaced femoral neck fractures (DFNFs) has also been understood to be a risk factor for instability. In our study, THA procedures were reported as either elective or non-elective procedures, with the assumption that non-elective surgery was performed secondary to DFNFs in most instances. Our results suggest that elective surgery confers 86% less likelihood of sustaining an in-hospital dislocation when compared to surgery for a DFNF. This is in agreement with the literature with the reported overall dislocation rates ranging from 6% to 20%, significantly higher than primary THA for osteoarthritis (OA) [17,21].

Our data imply that Parkinson's patients have a 93% greater odds of sustaining an in-hospital dislocation, which is in agreement with the prior literature with the overall rates of dislocation reported to be as high as 4 to 7% [17]. This likely relates to neuromuscular control and may be especially important in the immediate postoperative period during early mobilization.

SLE also was found to be a significant risk factor for early dislocation in our study. This is in agreement with the literature, which tends to focus on inflammatory arthritis as a whole [17,22]. In a database study by Viswanathan et al., the rate of dislocation in SLE patients was 2.6% compared to 1.4% in non-SLE patients [23], which would agree with our findings, with soft tissue differences once again hypothesized to be the culprit.

Given the elevated risks that these factors impose, it may be prudent to consider these during postoperative management with differing range-of-motion restrictions, use of abduction pillow orthoses, etc. It may also be useful to consider during surgical planning with implant selection (e.g., larger femoral heads, cup positioning, use of dual mobility design, modular components) and/or decision to perform soft tissue repair on patients with several of these major risk factors.

Early dislocation remains a challenging issue and a large financial burden on the healthcare system. We were able to show that an in-hospital dislocation increases the average cost of a THA by nearly USD 34,000 and more than doubles the length of stay. This also does not account for the cost associated with disposition after discharge from the hospital.

We do acknowledge several limitations in our study design. First, we acknowledge our retrospective study design, as well as collecting data from multiple centers, multiple surgeons, and different postoperative protocols. Second, we do acknowledge the limits of the NIS database, which is based on ICD-10 codes and carries the potential to limit data collection. The NIS also does not report on the duration of each procedure, implant selection or positioning, ambulation delays postoperatively, or skill level of the surgeon operating (attending, fellow, resident, etc.); therefore, their potential effects on in-hospital dislocation could not be included in this study. However, our study is strengthened by the comprehensive nature of the NIS database, including a large, national sample size as well as the inclusion of more urgent THA cases.

5. Conclusions

With the projected increase in THA volume over the coming decade, there is an increased necessity to identify risk factors for adverse events such as early THA dislocation, particularly in the immediate postoperative period. This study identified older age, female sex, SLE, and Parkinson's disease as risk factors for early in-hospital dislocation, while elective surgery appeared to decrease risk. These findings can be used as a basis for further research in the field as well as help surgeons implement preventative strategies in these patients who are at high risk irrespective of their experience or technique. Additionally, our findings highlight the financial burden of this problem and can help healthcare policy makers understand the impact that these factors have on healthcare facilities.

Author Contributions: Conceptualization, H.B.J., A.J.H., Y.L., and S.N.S. methodology, H.B.J. and S.N.S.; software, S.N.S.; validation, H.B.J., A.J.H., and S.N.S.; formal analysis, H.B.J. and S.N.S.; investigation, H.B.J. and S.N.S.; data curation, H.B.J. and S.N.S.; writing—original draft preparation, H.B.J.; writing—review and editing, H.B.J., A.J.H., Y.L., and S.N.S.; supervision, S.N.S. All authors have read and agreed to the published version of the manuscript.

Funding: This research received no external funding.

Institutional Review Board Statement: All procedures were performed in compliance with the relevant laws and institutional guidelines. This study was exempt from Institutional Review Board approval given the data are publicly available and de-identified.

Informed Consent Statement: Patient consent was waived due to the NIS database being publicly available and de-identified.

Data Availability Statement: The original data presented in this study are openly available in the NIS database, which can be found at https://hcup-us.ahrq.gov/db/nation/nis/nisdbdocumentation.jsp, accessed on 6 January 2023.

Acknowledgments: This research did not receive any specific grant from funding agencies in the public, commercial, or non-profit sectors.

Conflicts of Interest: The authors declare no financial conflicts of interest.

Appendix A

Table A1. ICD codes used.

THA		Obesity	Comorbidities	Periprosthetic Dislocation
0SR9019	0SRB0JA	E660	Diabetes without complications	T84020A
0SR901A	0SRB0JZ	E6601	E119	T84021A
0SR901Z	0SRB0KZ	E6609		T84022A
0SR9029	0SR90J9	E661	Diabetes with complications	T84023A
0SR902A	0SR90JA	E662	E1169	T84028A
0SR902Z	0SR90JZ	E668		T84029A
0SR9039	0SR90KZ	E669	Tobacco-related disorder	
0SR903A	0SRB019	Z6830	Z87891	
0SR903Z	0SRB01A	Z6831		
0SR9049	0SRB01Z	Z6832		
0SR904A	0SRB029	Z6833		
0SR904Z	0SRB02A	Z6834		
0SR9069	0SRB02Z	Z6835		
0SR906A	0SRB039	Z6836		
0SR906Z	0SRB03A	Z6837		
0SR907Z	0SRB03Z	Z6838		
0SR90EZ	0SRB049	Z6839		
0SRB06Z	0SRB04A			
0SRB07Z	0SRB04Z	Morbid obesity		
0SRB0EZ	0SRB069	Z6841		
0SRB0J9	0SRB06A	Z6842		
		Z6843		
		Z6844		
		Z6845		

References

1. Learmonth, I.D.; Young, C.; Rorabeck, C. The operation of the century: Total hip replacement. *Lancet* **2007**, *370*, 1508–1519. [CrossRef] [PubMed]
2. Shichman, I.; Roof, M.; Askew, N.; Nherera, L.; Rozell, J.C.; Seyler, T.M.; Schwarzkopf, R. Projections and Epidemiology of Primary Hip and Knee Arthroplasty in Medicare Patients to 2040–2060. *JB JS Open Access* **2023**, *8*, e22. [CrossRef] [PubMed]
3. Soong, M.; Rubash, H.E.; Macaulay, W. Dislocation after total hip arthroplasty. *J. Am. Acad. Orthop. Surg.* **2004**, *12*, 314–321. [CrossRef] [PubMed]
4. Bozic, K.J.; Kurtz, S.M.; Lau, E.; Ong, K.; Vail, T.P.; Berry, D.J. The epidemiology of revision total hip arthroplasty in the United States. *J. Bone Jt. Surg. Am.* **2009**, *91*, 128–133. [CrossRef] [PubMed]
5. Gwam, C.U.; Mistry, J.B.; Mohamed, N.S.; Thomas, M.; Bigart, K.C.; Mont, M.A.; Delanois, R.E. Current Epidemiology of Revision Total Hip Arthroplasty in the United States: National Inpatient Sample 2009 to 2013. *J. Arthroplast.* **2017**, *32*, 2088–2092. [CrossRef] [PubMed]
6. Falez, F.; Papalia, M.; Favetti, F.; Panegrossi, G.; Casella, F.; Mazzotta, G. Total hip arthroplasty instability in Italy. *Int. Orthop.* **2017**, *41*, 635–644. [CrossRef] [PubMed]
7. Pieringer, H.; Labek, G.; Auersperg, V.; Böhler, N. Cementless total hip arthroplasty in patients older than 80 years of age. *J. Bone Jt. Surg. Br.* **2003**, *85*, 641–645. [CrossRef]
8. Ekelund, A.; Rydell, N.; Nilsson, O.S. Total hip arthroplasty in patients 80 years of age and older. *Clin. Orthop. Relat. Res.* **1992**, *281*, 101–106. [CrossRef]
9. Rowan, F.E.; Benjamin, B.; Pietrak, J.R.; Haddad, F.S. Prevention of Dislocation After Total Hip Arthroplasty. *J. Arthroplast.* **2018**, *33*, 1316–1324. [CrossRef] [PubMed]
10. Weber, M.; Cabanela, M.E.; Sim, F.H.; Frassica, F.J.; Harmsen, W.S. Total hip replacement in patients with Parkinson's disease. *Int. Orthop.* **2002**, *26*, 66–68.
11. Palan, J.; Beard, D.J.; Murray, D.W.; Andrew, J.G.; Nolan, J. Which approach for total hip arthroplasty: Anterolateral or posterior? *Clin. Orthop. Relat. Res.* **2009**, *467*, 473–477. [CrossRef] [PubMed]
12. Molloy, I.B.; Martin, B.I.; Moschetti, W.E.; Jevsevar, D.S. Effects of the Length of Stay on the Cost of Total Knee and Total Hip Arthroplasty from 2002 to 2013. *J. Bone Jt. Surg. Am.* **2017**, *99*, 402–407. [CrossRef] [PubMed]
13. Berry, D.J.; von Knoch, M.; Schleck, C.D.; Harmsen, W.S. The cumulative long-term risk of dislocation after primary Charnley total hip arthroplasty. *J. Bone Jt. Surg. Am.* **2004**, *86*, 9–14. [CrossRef] [PubMed]

14. Gausden, E.B.; Parhar, H.S.; Popper, J.E.; Sculco, P.K.; Rush, B.N.M. Risk Factors for Early Dislocation Following Primary Elective Total Hip Arthroplasty. *J. Arthroplast.* **2018**, *33*, 1567–1571.e2. [CrossRef] [PubMed]
15. Goel, A.; Lau, E.C.; Ong, K.L.; Berry, D.J.; Malkani, A.L. Dislocation rates following primary total hip arthroplasty have plateaued in the Medicare population. *J. Arthroplast.* **2015**, *30*, 743–746. [CrossRef] [PubMed]
16. Hermansen, L.L.; Viberg, B.; Overgaard, S. Large hospital variation in the risk of dislocation after primary total hip arthroplasty for primary osteoarthritis: 31,105 patients in 59 hospitals from the Danish Hip Arthroplasty Register. *Acta Orthop.* **2022**, *93*, 503–508. [CrossRef] [PubMed]
17. Meek, R.M.; Allan, D.B.; McPhillips, G.; Kerr, L.; Howie, C.R. Epidemiology of dislocation after total hip arthroplasty. *Clin. Orthop. Relat. Res.* **2006**, *447*, 9–18. [CrossRef] [PubMed]
18. Malkani, A.L.; Dilworth, B.; Ong, K.; Baykal, D.; Lau, E.; Mackin, T.N.; Lee, G.C. High Risk of Readmission in Octogenarians Undergoing Primary Hip Arthroplasty. *Clin. Orthop. Relat. Res.* **2017**, *475*, 2878–2888. [CrossRef] [PubMed]
19. Leichtle, U.G.; Leichtle, C.I.; Taslaci, F.; Reize, P.; Wünschel, M. Dislocation after total hip arthroplasty: Risk factors and treatment options. *Acta Orthop. Traumatol. Turc.* **2013**, *47*, 96–103. [CrossRef]
20. Mahomed, N.N.; Barrett, J.A.; Katz, J.N.; Phillips, C.B.; Losina, E.; Lew, R.A.; Guadagnoli, E.; Harris, W.H.; Poss, R.; Baron, J.A. Rates and outcomes of primary and revision total hip replacement in the United States medicare population. *J. Bone Jt. Surg. Am.* **2003**, *85*, 27–32. [CrossRef]
21. Noticewala, M.; Murtaugh, T.S.; Danoff, J.; Cunn, G.J.; Shah, R.P.; Geller, J. Has the risk of dislocation after total hip arthroplasty performed for displaced femoral neck fracture improved with modern implants? *J. Clin. Orthop. Trauma.* **2018**, *9*, 281–284. [CrossRef] [PubMed]
22. Ravi, B.; Escott, B.; Shah, P.S.; Jenkinson, R.; Chahal, J.; Bogoch, E.; Kreder, H.; Hawker, G. A systematic review and meta-analysis comparing complications following total joint arthroplasty for rheumatoid arthritis versus for osteoarthritis. *Arthritis Rheum.* **2012**, *64*, 3839–3849. [CrossRef] [PubMed]
23. Viswanathan, V.K.; Sakthivelnathan, V.; Senthil, T.; Menedal, A.; Purudappa, P.P.; Mounasamy, V.; Sambandam, S. Does systemic lupus erythematosus impact the peri-operative complication rates following primary total knee arthroplasty? A national inpatient sample-based large-scale study. *Arch. Orthop. Trauma. Surg.* **2023**, *143*, 3291–3298. [CrossRef] [PubMed]

Disclaimer/Publisher's Note: The statements, opinions and data contained in all publications are solely those of the individual author(s) and contributor(s) and not of MDPI and/or the editor(s). MDPI and/or the editor(s) disclaim responsibility for any injury to people or property resulting from any ideas, methods, instructions or products referred to in the content.

Appendix A

Table A1. ICD codes used.

THA		Obesity	Comorbidities	Periprosthetic Dislocation
0SR9019	0SRB0JA	E660	Diabetes without complications	T84020A
0SR901A	0SRB0JZ	E6601	E119	T84021A
0SR901Z	0SRB0KZ	E6609		T84022A
0SR9029	0SR90J9	E661	Diabetes with complications	T84023A
0SR902A	0SR90JA	E662	E1169	T84028A
0SR902Z	0SR90JZ	E668		T84029A
0SR9039	0SR90KZ	E669	Tobacco-related disorder	
0SR903A	0SRB019	Z6830	Z87891	
0SR903Z	0SRB01A	Z6831		
0SR9049	0SRB01Z	Z6832		
0SR904A	0SRB029	Z6833		
0SR904Z	0SRB02A	Z6834		
0SR9069	0SRB02Z	Z6835		
0SR906A	0SRB039	Z6836		
0SR906Z	0SRB03A	Z6837		
0SR907Z	0SRB03Z	Z6838		
0SR90EZ	0SRB049	Z6839		
0SRB06Z	0SRB04A			
0SRB07Z	0SRB04Z	Morbid obesity		
0SRB0EZ	0SRB069	Z6841		
0SRB0J9	0SRB06A	Z6842		
		Z6843		
		Z6844		
		Z6845		

References

1. Learmonth, I.D.; Young, C.; Rorabeck, C. The operation of the century: Total hip replacement. *Lancet* **2007**, *370*, 1508–1519. [CrossRef] [PubMed]
2. Shichman, I.; Roof, M.; Askew, N.; Nherera, L.; Rozell, J.C.; Seyler, T.M.; Schwarzkopf, R. Projections and Epidemiology of Primary Hip and Knee Arthroplasty in Medicare Patients to 2040–2060. *JB JS Open Access* **2023**, *8*, e22. [CrossRef] [PubMed]
3. Soong, M.; Rubash, H.E.; Macaulay, W. Dislocation after total hip arthroplasty. *J. Am. Acad. Orthop. Surg.* **2004**, *12*, 314–321. [CrossRef] [PubMed]
4. Bozic, K.J.; Kurtz, S.M.; Lau, E.; Ong, K.; Vail, T.P.; Berry, D.J. The epidemiology of revision total hip arthroplasty in the United States. *J. Bone Jt. Surg. Am.* **2009**, *91*, 128–133. [CrossRef] [PubMed]
5. Gwam, C.U.; Mistry, J.B.; Mohamed, N.S.; Thomas, M.; Bigart, K.C.; Mont, M.A.; Delanois, R.E. Current Epidemiology of Revision Total Hip Arthroplasty in the United States: National Inpatient Sample 2009 to 2013. *J. Arthroplast.* **2017**, *32*, 2088–2092. [CrossRef] [PubMed]
6. Falez, F.; Papalia, M.; Favetti, F.; Panegrossi, G.; Casella, F.; Mazzotta, G. Total hip arthroplasty instability in Italy. *Int. Orthop.* **2017**, *41*, 635–644. [CrossRef] [PubMed]
7. Pieringer, H.; Labek, G.; Auersperg, V.; Böhler, N. Cementless total hip arthroplasty in patients older than 80 years of age. *J. Bone Jt. Surg. Br.* **2003**, *85*, 641–645. [CrossRef]
8. Ekelund, A.; Rydell, N.; Nilsson, O.S. Total hip arthroplasty in patients 80 years of age and older. *Clin. Orthop. Relat. Res.* **1992**, *281*, 101–106. [CrossRef]
9. Rowan, F.E.; Benjamin, B.; Pietrak, J.R.; Haddad, F.S. Prevention of Dislocation After Total Hip Arthroplasty. *J. Arthroplast.* **2018**, *33*, 1316–1324. [CrossRef] [PubMed]
10. Weber, M.; Cabanela, M.E.; Sim, F.H.; Frassica, F.J.; Harmsen, W.S. Total hip replacement in patients with Parkinson's disease. *Int. Orthop.* **2002**, *26*, 66–68.
11. Palan, J.; Beard, D.J.; Murray, D.W.; Andrew, J.G.; Nolan, J. Which approach for total hip arthroplasty: Anterolateral or posterior? *Clin. Orthop. Relat. Res.* **2009**, *467*, 473–477. [CrossRef] [PubMed]
12. Molloy, I.B.; Martin, B.I.; Moschetti, W.E.; Jevsevar, D.S. Effects of the Length of Stay on the Cost of Total Knee and Total Hip Arthroplasty from 2002 to 2013. *J. Bone Jt. Surg. Am.* **2017**, *99*, 402–407. [CrossRef] [PubMed]
13. Berry, D.J.; von Knoch, M.; Schleck, C.D.; Harmsen, W.S. The cumulative long-term risk of dislocation after primary Charnley total hip arthroplasty. *J. Bone Jt. Surg. Am.* **2004**, *86*, 9–14. [CrossRef] [PubMed]

14. Gausden, E.B.; Parhar, H.S.; Popper, J.E.; Sculco, P.K.; Rush, B.N.M. Risk Factors for Early Dislocation Following Primary Elective Total Hip Arthroplasty. *J. Arthroplast.* **2018**, *33*, 1567–1571.e2. [CrossRef] [PubMed]
15. Goel, A.; Lau, E.C.; Ong, K.L.; Berry, D.J.; Malkani, A.L. Dislocation rates following primary total hip arthroplasty have plateaued in the Medicare population. *J. Arthroplast.* **2015**, *30*, 743–746. [CrossRef] [PubMed]
16. Hermansen, L.L.; Viberg, B.; Overgaard, S. Large hospital variation in the risk of dislocation after primary total hip arthroplasty for primary osteoarthritis: 31,105 patients in 59 hospitals from the Danish Hip Arthroplasty Register. *Acta Orthop.* **2022**, *93*, 503–508. [CrossRef] [PubMed]
17. Meek, R.M.; Allan, D.B.; McPhillips, G.; Kerr, L.; Howie, C.R. Epidemiology of dislocation after total hip arthroplasty. *Clin. Orthop. Relat. Res.* **2006**, *447*, 9–18. [CrossRef] [PubMed]
18. Malkani, A.L.; Dilworth, B.; Ong, K.; Baykal, D.; Lau, E.; Mackin, T.N.; Lee, G.C. High Risk of Readmission in Octogenarians Undergoing Primary Hip Arthroplasty. *Clin. Orthop. Relat. Res.* **2017**, *475*, 2878–2888. [CrossRef] [PubMed]
19. Leichtle, U.G.; Leichtle, C.I.; Taslaci, F.; Reize, P.; Wünschel, M. Dislocation after total hip arthroplasty: Risk factors and treatment options. *Acta Orthop. Traumatol. Turc.* **2013**, *47*, 96–103. [CrossRef]
20. Mahomed, N.N.; Barrett, J.A.; Katz, J.N.; Phillips, C.B.; Losina, E.; Lew, R.A.; Guadagnoli, E.; Harris, W.H.; Poss, R.; Baron, J.A. Rates and outcomes of primary and revision total hip replacement in the United States medicare population. *J. Bone Jt. Surg. Am.* **2003**, *85*, 27–32. [CrossRef]
21. Noticewala, M.; Murtaugh, T.S.; Danoff, J.; Cunn, G.J.; Shah, R.P.; Geller, J. Has the risk of dislocation after total hip arthroplasty performed for displaced femoral neck fracture improved with modern implants? *J. Clin. Orthop. Trauma.* **2018**, *9*, 281–284. [CrossRef] [PubMed]
22. Ravi, B.; Escott, B.; Shah, P.S.; Jenkinson, R.; Chahal, J.; Bogoch, E.; Kreder, H.; Hawker, G. A systematic review and meta-analysis comparing complications following total joint arthroplasty for rheumatoid arthritis versus for osteoarthritis. *Arthritis Rheum.* **2012**, *64*, 3839–3849. [CrossRef] [PubMed]
23. Viswanathan, V.K.; Sakthivelnathan, V.; Senthil, T.; Menedal, A.; Purudappa, P.P.; Mounasamy, V.; Sambandam, S. Does systemic lupus erythematosus impact the peri-operative complication rates following primary total knee arthroplasty? A national inpatient sample-based large-scale study. *Arch. Orthop. Trauma. Surg.* **2023**, *143*, 3291–3298. [CrossRef] [PubMed]

Disclaimer/Publisher's Note: The statements, opinions and data contained in all publications are solely those of the individual author(s) and contributor(s) and not of MDPI and/or the editor(s). MDPI and/or the editor(s) disclaim responsibility for any injury to people or property resulting from any ideas, methods, instructions or products referred to in the content.

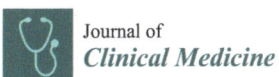

Article

Comparison of Five-Day vs. Fourteen-Day Incubation of Cultures for Diagnosis of Periprosthetic Joint Infection in Hip Arthroplasty

Catalina Baez [1,*], Robert MacDonell [1], Abtahi Tishad [2], Hernan A. Prieto [1], Emilie N. Miley [1], Justin T. Deen [3], Chancellor F. Gray [3], Hari K. Parvataneni [3] and Luis Pulido [3,*]

1 Department of Orthopaedic Surgery and Sports Medicine, University of Florida, Gainesville, FL 32607, USA; rtmacdonell@gmail.com (R.M.); prieth@ortho.ufl.edu (H.A.P.); emilie.miley1@gmail.com (E.N.M.)
2 College of Medicine, University of Florida, Gainesville, FL 32607, USA; tishad100@ufl.edu
3 Florida Orthopaedic Institute, Gainesville, FL 32607, USA; deenju812@gmail.com (J.T.D.); chancellor.gray@gmail.com (C.F.G.); hkparvataneni@gmail.com (H.K.P.)
* Correspondence: baezc@ortho.ufl.edu (C.B.); luispulidos@yahoo.com (L.P.)

Abstract: Background: Periprosthetic joint infections (PJI) are among the most morbid complications in total hip arthroplasty (THA). The ideal incubation time, however, for intraoperative cultures for PJI diagnosis remains unclear. As such, the aim of this study was to determine if any differences existed in culture-positive rates and organism detection between five-day and fourteen-day cultures. **Methods:** This retrospective cohort study consisted of THA cases diagnosed with PJI performed between May 2014 and May 2020 at a single tertiary-care institution. Analyses compared five-day and fourteen-day cultures and carried out a pre-specified subgroup analysis by organism and PJI type. **Results:** A total of 147 surgeries were performed in 101 patients (57.1% females), of which 65% (n = 98) obtained five-day cultures and 34% (n = 49) obtained fourteen-day cultures. The positive culture rate was 67.3% (n = 99) with *Staphylococcus aureus* being the most common pathogen identified (n = 41 specimens, 41.4%). The positive culture rate was not significantly different between groups (66.3% five-day, 69.4% fourteen-day, $p = 0.852$). Fourteen-day cultures had a significantly longer time-to-positive culture (5.0 days) than five-day cultures (3.0 days, $p < 0.001$), a higher rate of fungi (5.6% vs. 0%), and a lower rate of Gram-negatives (4.5% vs. 18.7%, $p = 0.016$). **Conclusions:** Fourteen-day cultures did not increase the positivity rate, had higher rates of slow-growth pathogens, and had a longer time-to-positivization than five-day cultures. Prolonged culture holds may provide more thorough organism detection for PJI without increasing the diagnostic culture yield.

Keywords: prosthetic joint infection; total hip arthroplasty; intraoperative cultures; culture hold times

1. Introduction

Prosthetic joint infections (PJI) have a seemingly sparse incidence of 0.76% to 1.24% [1]. However, they are associated with significant morbidity, causing severe psychological [2] and economic [3] burden on the patient, including mortality, with death rates increasing progressively following revision arthroplasty from 5.5 to 8% (1-year postoperative), 11 to 25% (2-years postoperative), and 40 to 45% (5-years postoperative) [4–7]. In addition, there has been a 2.6-fold increase in annual procedures performed for PJI treatment between 2006 and 2013 [8]. The yearly cost of these procedures exceeded USD 500 million in 2017 and is expected to increase to USD 753.4 million by 2030 [9] as the annual volume of total hip arthroplasty (THA) surgery will increase by 174% by 2030 [1]. This historical increase in the incidence of PJI cases highlights the need for clinicians and researchers to determine the best approach to diagnose PJI.

Released in 2018, the revised Musculoskeletal Infection Society (MSIS) criteria uses a scoring system based on a combination of culture, laboratory, and clinical presentation findings to yield a diagnosis with 99.7% sensitivity and 99.5% specificity [10]. A major criterion for diagnosis is the isolation of a single organism in two separate cultures of periprosthetic tissue or synovial fluid [10]. However, a lack of literature exists to determine the ideal culture time for periprosthetic tissue samples as it appears highly organism-dependent [11–15] with wide variation in incubation times for anaerobic and aerobic samples [16]. A 2018 study demonstrated that while most infected samples yielded positive culture results within five days, some samples (i.e., *Cutibacterium acnes* (*C. acnes*)) needed ten or more days to yield positive culture results [11]. Previous PJI diagnosis and management guidelines have failed to address recommendations on the ideal culture incubation duration [10,17,18], and historical trends have proposed culture incubation durations varying from four to fourteen days [12,17].

Considering these inconsistencies in the literature, the aim of this study was to determine if there was a difference in positivity rates, organism growth, time of growth, treatment, and disease-free survival between five-day and fourteen-day cultures in THA PJI. Additionally, we sought to determine the organism profile for PJI in our tertiary-care institution and whether there is an association between preoperative Synovasure® (Zimmer Biomet, Warsaw, IN, USA) synovial fluid cultures and intraoperative culture organism characterization performed at our hospital laboratory.

2. Materials and Methods

After obtaining Institutional Review Board approval, a retrospective cohort study was performed on THA patients diagnosed with PJI from May 2014 through May 2020. Our hospital laboratory transitioned culture hold times in May 2018. Before this time, all cultures were held for five days. Following this transition, cultures were held for fourteen days. All findings from this study are reported following the Strengthening the Reporting of Observational Studies in Epidemiology (STROBE) guidelines [19].

2.1. Participants

The inclusion criteria were THA cases with a diagnosis and treatment for PJI that underwent revision surgery and intraoperative cultures were obtained (CPT codes: 27134, 27137, 27138, 27091, 20680, 11981, 20702, 10061). We included only patients with a minimum one-year follow-up visit. The diagnosis of PJI was based on the 2018 revised MSIS criteria [10]. We excluded all cases where PJI diagnostic criteria were not met, subjects for which intraoperative cultures were not obtained, and patients with less than one-year follow-up.

2.2. Variables and Outcome Measures

Demographic data, including patient medical history (i.e., age, body mass index (BMI), sex), comorbidities (i.e., smoking status, diabetes mellitus (DM)), and PJI data were collected for this study via chart review of the electronic medical record. In addition, perioperative, operative, and postoperative data, surgical and antibiotic treatment, and complications reported during the first year following surgery were collected. Given that the culture hold time was the same for all specimens obtained during each surgery, we compared outcomes across five-day and fourteen-day culture holds by grouping all intraoperative culture specimens into one surgical culture sample (i.e., if one or more of the specimens obtained intraoperatively were positive, this surgical case was determined to be a culture-positive case) for statistical analysis. All organism-specific data were compared using individual culture specimen data for those that reported microbial growth. Thus, the number of intraoperative specimens sent in for culture, the number of specimens that were positive for microbial growth, the time to positive culture, organisms reported, antibiotic selection, definitive surgical intervention (i.e., debridement, antibiotics and implant retention (DAIR), one-stage revision, two-stage revision, resection arthroplasty, and amputation), surgical treatment failure, and disease-free survival were compared using the grouped surgical culture sample data. We defined surgical treatment failure according to the MSIS 2018 consensus [20], where Tiers 3 and 4 represent surgical treatment failure. Disease-free survival was defined as the total follow-up time without further PJI management.

The time to positive culture by organism, type of PJI (i.e., early postoperative, acute hematogenous, and chronic), surgical treatment failure, and complications during the first year after surgery (i.e., readmissions in the first 30 days postoperative and death in the first 365 days postoperative) were obtained to define the PJI organism profile for this institution. Finally, Synovasure® culture reports were collected to compare with intraoperative culture organisms.

2.3. Statistical Analysis

Statistical analyses were performed using the statistical software IBM SPSS Version 28. Categorical measures were summarized as counts (n) and percentages (%), and continuous measures were summarized as means and standard deviations (SD). Categorical variables were analyzed for between-group comparisons with chi-square and Fisher's exact tests. Given the non-normal characteristics of the data, the Kruskal–Wallis test was used to compare continuous data. Survival analyses were performed using Kaplan–Meier curves and the log-rank test for between-group comparisons. Prespecified subgroup analyses were completed for low-virulence organisms (i.e., C. acnes, Cutibacterium albicans (C. albicans), mycobacteria, and anaerobes) and different organism types (i.e., Gram-positive, Gram-negative, anaerobes, fungi). Disease-free survival was defined as the total follow-up time without further PJI management, and case censoring was defined as surgical treatment failure according to the MSIS 2018 consensus [10]. Statistical significance was predefined at a $p < 0.05$.

3. Results

A total of 147 surgeries were identified for 101 patients with a PJI diagnosis from May 2014 to May 2020. Of these, 66.7% (n = 98) of the surgical culture samples were held for five days, and 33.3% (n = 49) were held for fourteen days. In total, 57.1% (n = 84) were male, and 63% (n = 42.9) were female, with a mean age of 62.0 (±12.7) years and a mean BMI of 30.8 (±9.0). A total of 19% (n = 28) of the patients in the sample reported being active smokers at the time of PJI diagnosis, and 32% (n = 47) had a diagnosis of diabetes mellitus (DM). The McPherson host grade [21] rates were 12.2% (n = 18) grade A, 46.3% (n = 68) grade B, and 41.5% (n = 61) grade C. Additionally, 71.4% (n = 105) of cases were classified as chronic PJI, 15.6% (n = 23) as acute hematogenous, and 12.9% (n = 19) as early postoperative. No significant differences were identified for patient demographics between the five-day and fourteen-day groups (Table 1).

Table 1. Patient demographics.

	Total N = 147	5-Day Cultures N = 98	14-Day Cultures N = 49	p-Value
Age, mean (SD)	62.0 (12.7)	61.5 (12.1)	61.4 (12.7)	0.976
BMI, mean (SD)	30.8 (9.1)	30.2 (8.8)	31.2 (7.6)	0.612
Sex, n (%)				0.216
Female	63 (42.9)	38 (38.8)	25 (51.0)	
Male	84 (57.1)	60 (61.2)	24 (49.0)	
McPherson Host Grade, n (%)				0.249
A	18 (12.2)	15 (15.3)	3 (6.1)	
B	68 (46.3)	45 (45.9)	23 (46.9)	
C	61 (41.5)	38 (38.8)	23 (46.9)	
Active Smoking, n (%)	28 (19.0)	20 (20.4)	8 (16.3)	0.710
DM, n (%)	47 (32.0)	33 (33.7)	14 (28.6)	0.662
Laterality, n (%)				0.600
Left	72 (49.0)	46 (46.9)	26 (53.1)	
Right	75 (51.0)	52 (53.1)	23 (46.9)	
Periprosthetic Joint Infection Type, n (%)				0.976
Early Postoperative	19 (12.9)	13 (13.3)	6 (12.2)	
Acute Hematogenous	23 (15.6)	15 (15.3)	8 (16.3)	
Chronic	105 (71.4)	70 (71.4)	35 (71.4)	

Abbreviations—BMI: body mass index; DM: diabetes mellitus type II.

3.1. Comparison of Five-Day and Fourteen-Day Cultures

The culture-positive rate for the full cohort was 67.3% (n = 99), with no significant differences between five-day and fourteen-day cultures ($p = 0.852$, Table 2). The mean number of individual specimens obtained during each surgery was 8.0 (± 4.2), of which a mean of 2.5 (± 1.4) specimens grew detectable organisms. There was no significant differences between five-day and fourteen-day cultures for the total number of specimens sent for culture ($p = 0.079$) or the number of positive specimens ($p = 0.527$, Table 2).

Table 2. Comparison between 5-day and 14-day cultures.

	Total N = 147	5-Day Cultures N = 98	14-Day Cultures N = 49	*p*-Value
Culture Positive Rate, n (%)	99 (67.3)	65 (66.3)	34 (69.4)	0.852
Intraoperative Specimens, Mean (SD)	8.0 (4.2)	8.3 (3.9)	7.6 (4.9)	0.079
Positive Specimens, Mean (SD)	2.5 (1.4)	2.6 (1.5)	2.4 (1.4)	0.527
Time to Positive Culture, Median (Range)	4.0 (0–23)	3.0 (0–7)	5.0 (0–23)	**<0.001**
Colonization, n (%)				0.135
Monomicrobial	82 (82.2)	57 (87.7)	25 (73.5)	
Polymicrobial	17 (17.2)	8 (12.3)	9 (26.5)	
S. aureus sensitivities, n (%)				0.541
MRSA	20 (48.8)	16 (53.3)	4 (36.4)	
MSSA	21 (51.2)	14 (46.7)	7 (63.6)	
Organism Type, n (%)				**0.016**
Gram-Positive	100 (84.0)	60 (80.0)	40 (90.9)	
Gram-Negative	16 (13.4)	14 (18.7)	2 (4.5)	
Anaerobe	1 (0.8)	1 (1.3)	0 (0.0)	
Fungi	2 (1.7)	0 (0.0)	2 (4.5)	
Definitive Surgery, n (%)				0.196
DAIR	24 (16.3)	16 (16.3)	8 (16.3)	
1-Stage	33 (22.4)	18 (18.4)	15 (30.6)	
2-Stage	73 (49.7)	49 (50.0)	24 (49.0)	
Resection Arthroplasty	16 (10.9)	14 (14.3)	2 (4.1)	
Amputation	1 (0.7)	1 (1.0)	0 (0.0)	
Antibiotic Spectrum, n (%)				0.724
Narrow	8 (6.7)	6 (7.4)	2 (5.3)	
Broad	111 (93.3)	75 (92.6)	36 (94.7)	
Surgical Treatment Failure, n (%)	102 (69.4)	73 (71.6)	29 (28.4)	0.087

Abbreviations—MRSA: methicillin-resistant *Staphylococcus aureus*; MSSA: methicillin-sensitive *Staphylococcus aureus*; DAIR: debridement, antibiotics, and implant retention. Bolded: statistically significant.

The median time to positive culture was 4.0 days (range = 0–23 days). The time to positive culture was significantly longer for fourteen-day cultures with a median time of 5.0 days (range = 0–23 days), whereas the five-day cultures had a median of 3.0 days (range = 0–7 days, $p < 0.001$; Table 2). No significant differences were identified for the mono- and polymicrobial infections between five-day and fourteen-day cultures ($p = 0.135$; Table 2). Of the sample, *Staphylococcus aureus* (*S. aureus*) was the most detected organism, found in 34.4% (n = 41) of all positive specimens. Of these, methicillin-resistant *S. aureus* (MRSA) was present in 48.8% (n = 20) of the specimens, and methicillin-sensitive *S. aureus* (MSSA) was present in the remaining 51.2% (n = 21). No significant difference was identified between MRSA and MSSA rates between the five-day and fourteen-day cultures ($p = 0.541$; Table 2). However, the rates pertaining to the different types of organisms detected were significantly different between groups ($p = 0.016$; Table 2). Fungi were only detected in fourteen-day holds (4.5%, n = 2). Five-day holds had higher rates of Gram-negatives (18.7%, n = 14) and anaerobes (1.3%, n = 1). Gram-positives comprised the most common type of organism and were detected in both groups (Table 2).

The use of postoperative broad-spectrum antibiotics and culture-specific monotherapy was similar between the five-day and fourteen-day cultures ($p = 0.996$); additionally, definitive surgical management was also similar across groups ($p = 0.196$, Table 2). The surgical treatment failure rate was higher for the five-day cultures than for the fourteen-day cultures (74.5%, n = 73 vs. 59.2%, n = 29, respectively, $p = 0.087$), though not significantly different. Of these, 32.4% (n = 33) were reported in culture-negative cases and 67.6% (n = 69) in culture-positive cases. Kaplan–Meier survival curves reported a median disease-free survival of 226.0 weeks (95% CI: 106.9–345.1, Figure 1). The curve comparison using the log-rank test showed a significant difference between the survival curves for five-day and fourteen-day cultures ($p = 0.043$). Also, the median disease-free survival in the five-day cultures was 226.0 weeks (95% CI: 79.2–372.8) and it was 104.0 weeks in the fourteen-day cultures (95% CI: 65.2–142.8).

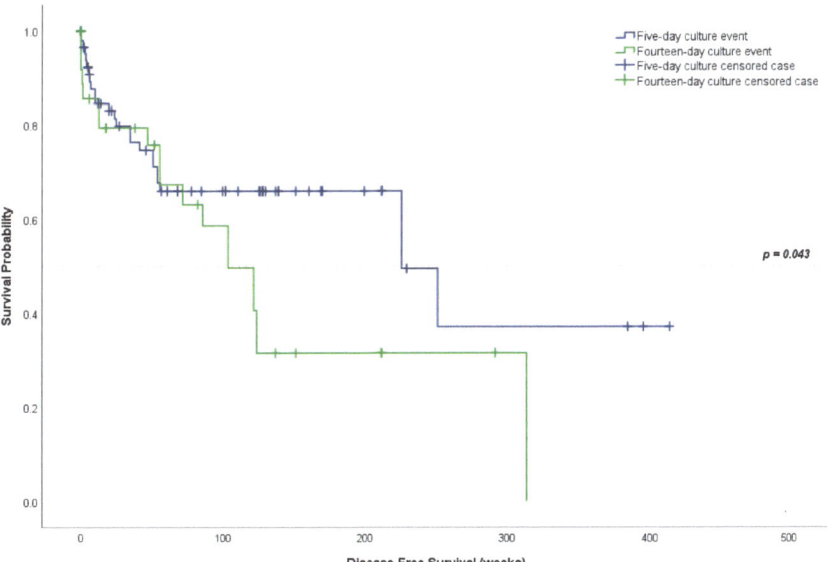

Figure 1. Kaplan–Meier curves for disease-free survival for five-day and fourteen-day culture cases.

3.2. Institutional Organism Profile

The time to positive culture by organism was significantly different, as *Trichosporon* sp. had the longest median time to positive (i.e., 23 days) and *Finegoldia magna* had the shortest (i.e., 0 days, $p = 0.011$). Subgroup analysis for low-virulence organisms demonstrated no significant difference between *C. acnes*, *C. albicans*, mycobacteria, and anaerobes ($p = 0.407$; Table 3). The time to positive culture by organism type was not statistically significant ($p = 0.063$; Table 3).

The rates of mono- and polymicrobial infections across PJI types were not significantly different ($p = 0.492$; Table 4). Additionally, the types of organism across types of PJI were not significantly different ($p = 0.312$; Table 4). However, surgical treatment failure was reported in 69.4% (n = 102) of cases. The comparison by PJI type was not statistically significant ($p = 0.107$), with chronic PJI in 76.5% (n = 78) of cases, acute hematogenous in 13.7% (n = 14) of cases, and early postoperative in 9.8% (n = 10; Table 5) of cases. When analyzed by the type of organism with mono- and polymicrobial infections, no significant differences were identified across the rates of surgical treatment failure ($p = 0.394$ and $p = 1.000$, respectively; Table 5).

Table 3. Comparison between 5-day and 14-day cultures.

	Individual Organism N (%)	Time to Positive Culture Median Days (Range)	p-Value
Organism Type (n = 119)			0.063
Gram-Positive	100 (84.0)	4.0 (0–11)	
Gram-Negative	16 (13.4)	3.5 (3–4)	
Anaerobes *	1 (0.8)	0.00 (0)	
Fungi	2 (1.7)	14.5 (6–23)	
Low Virulence Organisms (n = 8)			0.407
C. acnes	5 (4.2)	8.5 (2–11)	
C. albicans	1 (0.8)	6.0 (6)	
Mycobacteria **	1 (0.8)	7.0 (7)	
Anaerobes *	1 (0.8)	0.0 (0)	

* Only one obligate anaerobe was identified within the sample, *Finegoldia magna*, and was reported as positive in culture on the same day the sample was sent for culture. ** One type of mycobacteria was identified, *Mycobacteria fortuitum*, and *E. coli* was the only Gram-negative organism identified.

Table 4. Comparisons by PJI type.

	Total n (%)	Early Postoperative n (%)	Acute Hematogenous n (%)	Chronic n (%)	p-Value *
Colonization					0.492
Monomicrobial	82 (82.8)	14 (82.4)	16 (94.1)	52 (80.0)	
Polymicrobial	17 (17.2)	3 (17.6)	1 (5.9)	13 (20.0)	
Organism Type					0.250
Gram-Positive	100 (84.0)	17 (81.0)	11 (94.4)	66 (82.5)	
Gram-Negative	16 (13.4)	2 (9.5)	1 (5.6)	13 (16.3)	
Anaerobes	1 (0.8)	1 (4.8)	0 (0.0)	0 (0.0)	
Fungi	2 (1.7)	1 (4.8)	0 (0.0)	1 (1.3)	

Table 5. Complications and surgical treatment failure comparisons across PJI types.

	30-Day Readmissions n (%)	p-Value	365-Day Mortality n (%)	p-Value	Surgical Treatment Failure n (%)	p-Value
Colonization		1.000		0.315		1.000
Monomicrobial	17 (81.0)		1 (50.0)		57 (82.6)	
Polymicrobial	4 (19.0)		1 (50.0)		12 (17.4)	
Organism Type		0.114		0.180		0.394
Gram-Positive	19 (70.4)		2 (50.0)		65 (80.2)	
Gram-Negative	7 (25.9)		2 (50.0)		13 (16.0)	
Anaerobes	0 (0.0)		0 (0.0)		1 (1.2)	
Fungi	1 (3.7)		0 (0.0)		2 (2.5)	
PJI Type		0.360		1.000		0.107
Early Postoperative	3 (9.1)		0 (0.0)		10 (12.9)	
Acute Hematogenous	3 (9.1)		1 (33.3)		14 (13.7)	
Chronic	27 (81.8)		2 (66.7)		78 (76.5)	

Postoperative complication rates were compared across types of PJI, organisms, and colonization. Deaths during the first 365 days after surgery were reported in 2.0% of cases (n = 3). Comparison by PJI type was not statistically significant ($p = 1.000$), with chronic PJI identified in 66.7% (n = 2) of cases, followed by acute hematogenous in 33.3% (n = 1), and no reported deaths for early postoperative PJIs (Table 5). Similarly, when analyzed by the type of organism and mono- and polymicrobial infections, no significant differences were identified across mortality rates ($p = 0.080$ and $p = 0.315$, respectively, Table 5). Readmissions during the first 30 days after surgery were reported in 22.4% (n = 33) of cases. The comparison by organism type was statistically significant ($p = 0.050$), with Gram-positive organisms identified in 81.0% (n = 17) of cases, followed by Gram-negative organisms (4.8%, n = 1), fungi (4.8%, n = 1), and anaerobes (4.8%, n = 1). However, when analyzed by type of infection, organism, and mono- and polymicrobial infections, no significant differences were identified across readmission rates ($p = 0.360$, $p = 0.114$, and $p = 1.000$, respectively; Table 5).

3.3. Association of Synovial and Intraoperative Cultures

Preoperatively, 29.9% (n = 44) of cases had a Synovasure® test administered; of these, 70.5% (n = 31) reported negative organism detection, and the remaining 29.5% (n = 13) reported positive organism detection. However, no significant association existed between the organisms reported in Synovasure® testing and the intraoperative cultures ($p = 0.234$). Only six Synovasure® cases accurately reported the same organism found in intraoperative cultures. The congruently reported microorganisms in both tests were *S. agalactie*, MRSA, MSSA, coagulase-negative *S. aureus*, *S. epidermidis*, and *C. acnes*. The organisms that were reported in the intraoperative cultures but not in the preoperative Synovasure® testing were *E. faecium*, *Bacillus* sp., *Corynebacterium* sp., *E. coli*, *E. faecalis*, *K. pneumoniae*, *S. viridans*, and *C. albicans*.

4. Discussion

Our results demonstrated that fourteen-day cultures had a median growth time that was significantly longer and included higher rates of fungi detection than those held for five days. Previous literature has reported similar findings where other slow-growth organisms, like *C. acnes*, were detected during the second week of culture [12,22,23]. However, our findings show a median time to positive culture for *C. acnes* of 8.50 days (Table 3), further supporting the idea that shorter culture times potentially miss the diagnosis of slow-growing organisms.

Disease-free survival following surgical intervention for PJI was significantly longer for patients in the five-day culture group than in the fourteen-day culture group. However, the interpretation of these findings must consider lead-time bias, as the institutional shift from shorter to longer culture hold times was time-dependent. Patients in the fourteen-day cohort have yet to be followed long enough to deem this difference clinically significant. Our results failed to demonstrate a significant difference between culture hold times for the number of tissue samples sent for culture, the number of positive tissue samples, the rates of MRSA and MSSA, antibiotic coverage, and definitive surgical management of the PJI. Our findings reiterate those of Klement et al., who also failed to find a significant association between an improved surgical success of PJI treatment and more prolonged culture holds [15].

We found the culture positive rate to be similar across hold times, thus not increasing culture yield. This reiterates previous studies looking at similar comparisons [14,15]. However, it is important to note that other researchers have identified up to a 30% increase in positivity rate for longer culture times [12]. Previous literature, however, has reported concerns with the utility of longer culture times and the risk of an increased detection of contaminating organisms [12,14,15]. Although our results support previous findings on similar rates of polymicrobial infections across culture hold times [15], some organisms commonly categorized as contaminants [12,24] were identified in these polymicrobial cultures, primarily in those in the fourteen-day culture group. As such, there continues to be inconsistency regarding prolonged culture, which holds a risk of higher contamination rates as these organisms also have the potential for infection [12,24].

The most common organism detected in this sample was *S. aureus*, followed by coagulase-negative *Staphylococcus* species, which is consistent with epidemiological reports of PJI microbiology [13,25,26]. The time to positive culture was significantly different when compared by organism type; the largest difference was between fungi and Gram-negative organisms' growth time (Table 3). However, this finding was not the case for low virulence organisms; the median growth time identified for this subgroup was 6.14 days. Both of these findings underscore the potential effect of prolonged culture holds. Significant differences in growth time between commonly slow-growing organisms (e.g., fungi) and faster-growing organisms (e.g., Gram-negatives), and the similarity among organisms considered "low virulence" point to more extended culture holds, allowing for sufficient time to detect these organisms in a sample [12,27].

Our cohort's surgical treatment failure rate was higher than other rates reported in the literature [28–30]. However, there is inconsistency regarding the definition of treatment failure present in these studies. Most treatment failure cases were in the five-day culture group, with one-third of failures reported in culture-negative cases. These findings underscore the significance of determining the best available culture hold time. In our study, subgroup analyses did not reveal significant differences across PJI types, organism, and colonization types, which is also supported by previous research that has identified no association between the organism and colonization type and failure rates [31].

Finally, no significant association was identified between the organisms reported from intraoperative cultures and Synovasure® cultures, with only six cases accurately reporting the same organism in both cultures. However, Synovasure® testing reported negative culture results in multiple cases where intraoperative cultures reported organisms commonly qualified as contaminants. This descriptive trend in the data highlights the potential for the culture overgrowth of environmental contaminants, a common pitfall in extended bacterial culture sampling [12,24]. However, clinicians must be mindful that common culture contaminants can also overgrow and cause PJI, regardless of their categorization [12]. Thus, the correlation between intraoperative culture, Synovasure® results, and clinical and laboratory findings is imperative when determining diagnosis, management, and antibiotic coverage [10]. Our findings are echoed by a previous systematic review that identified variable concordance between Synovasure® and intraoperative cultures [32]. Previous research in this institution has supported the use of the Synovasure® test's alpha-defensin levels to have high sensitivity in PJI diagnosis and specificity following two-stage reimplantation [33,34]. However, further research is necessary to evaluate the role of Synovasure® cultures compared to intraoperative cultures. It remains unclear if there is any association between these results and the length of intraoperative culture hold, as this was not the goal of this study.

The results must be interpreted considering the limitations of this study. First, the retrospective nature of this study introduces an opportunity for selection and lead-time bias. This limitation becomes more important for disease-free survival comparisons, with five-day cultures being the standard of care during the first four years of data collection and fourteen-day cultures for the last two years of data collection. Patients who were diagnosed using five-day cultures were inherently followed for a longer period than the fourteen-day culture patients. Second, there was a relatively small sample size of 147 surgical culture samples for analysis. However, given that this study aimed to analyze outcomes from an uncommon, but impactful, complication of total joint arthroplasty, this sample size and methodology are justifiable and comparable to similar studies. Third, there was an unbalanced sample size between five-day and fourteen-day cultures. Although this distribution of samples was expected due to the period analyzed, this imbalance may impact the study's statistical power. However, in findings where statistical significance was identified to favor the fourteen-day cultures, this 2:1 sample distribution underscores the meaningfulness of these differences. Fourth, as this study was performed at a single institution, this may limit the generalizability of the results. However, surgeries were performed by eight different fellowship-trained arthroplasty surgeons, introducing variability into the dataset and expanding the applicability of the results. Future research should focus on longer culture holds and sensitivity and specificity regarding contaminant organism detection. Similarly, investigation into the cost-effectiveness of longer culture holds and the potential impact on accurate organism detection and PJI management is needed, as it becomes increasingly clear that there continues to be potential benefits in longer culture holds.

5. Conclusions

This retrospective cohort study revealed that fourteen-day cultures did not increase the positivity rate, rate of polymicrobial infections, or number of positive specimens reported, and it also identified a similar disease-free survival to five-day cultures. Fourteen-day culture holds demonstrated higher fungi growth rates and a longer time-to-positivization than five-day cultures. More prolonged culture holds may provide a more thorough organism detection for PJI; however, the risk of contaminant over-detection remains. In light of these findings, arthroplasty surgeons should consider increasing intraoperative culture hold times to fourteen days due to the potential for the increased detection of low-virulence organisms known for introducing complexity to managing PJI cases.

Author Contributions: Conceptualization, C.B., L.P. and R.M.; methodology C.B., L.P. and R.M.; software, C.B.; validation, C.B., A.T. and R.M.; formal analysis, C.B.; investigation, C.B., L.P. and R.M.; data curation, C.B., A.T. and R.M.; writing—original draft preparation, C.B., A.T. and L.P.; writing—review and editing, H.A.P., E.N.M., J.T.D., C.F.G., H.K.P. and L.P.; supervision, L.P.; project administration, E.N.M. All authors have read and agreed to the published version of the manuscript.

Funding: This research received no external funding.

Institutional Review Board Statement: The study was conducted in accordance with the Declaration of Helsinki and approved by the Institutional Review Board of University of Florida IRB202001322 approved on 15 June 2020.

Informed Consent Statement: Patient consent was waived due to this study being a retrospective chart review.

Data Availability Statement: The dataset analyzed during the study are not publicly available per study protocol. De-identified data may be available from the corresponding author with permission from the University of Florida upon reasonable request.

Conflicts of Interest: The authors declare no conflicts of interest.

References

1. Springer, B.D.; Cahue, S.; Etkin, C.D.; Lewallen, D.G.; McGrory, B.J. Infection burden in total hip and knee arthroplasties: An international registry-based perspective. *Arthroplast. Today* **2017**, *3*, 137–140. [CrossRef]
2. Andersson, A.E.; Bergh, I.; Karlsson, J.; Nilsson, K. Patients' experiences of acquiring a deep surgical site infection: An interview study. *Am. J. Infect. Control* **2010**, *38*, 711–717. [CrossRef]
3. Kurtz, S.M.; Lau, E.; Watson, H.; Schmier, J.K.; Parvizi, J. Economic burden of periprosthetic joint infection in the United States. *J. Arthroplast.* **2012**, *27*, 61–65.e1. [CrossRef] [PubMed]
4. Zmistowski, B.; Karam, J.A.; Durinka, J.B.; Casper, D.S.; Parvizi, J. Periprosthetic joint infection increases the risk of one-year mortality. *J. Bone Jt. Surg. Am.* **2013**, *95*, 2177–2184. [CrossRef] [PubMed]
5. Petis, S.M.; Abdel, M.P.; Perry, K.I.; Mabry, T.M.; Hanssen, A.D.; Berry, D.J. Long-Term Results of a 2-Stage Exchange Protocol for Periprosthetic Joint Infection Following Total Hip Arthroplasty in 164 Hips. *J. Bone Jt. Surg. Am.* **2019**, *101*, 74–84. [CrossRef]
6. Kildow, B.J.; Springer, B.D.; Brown, T.S.; Lyden, E.; Fehring, T.K.; Garvin, K.L. Long Term Results of Two-Stage Revision for Chronic Periprosthetic Hip Infection: A Multicenter Study. *J. Clin. Med.* **2022**, *11*, 1657. [CrossRef] [PubMed]
7. Fischbacher, A.; Borens, O. Prosthetic-joint Infections: Mortality Over the Last 10 Years. *J. Bone Jt. Infect.* **2019**, *4*, 198–202. [CrossRef] [PubMed]
8. Lenguerrand, E.; Whitehouse, M.R.; Beswick, A.D.; Jones, S.A.; Porter, M.L.; Blom, A.W. Revision for prosthetic joint infection following hip arthroplasty: Evidence from the National Joint Registry. *Bone Jt. Res.* **2017**, *6*, 391–398. [CrossRef]
9. Premkumar, A.; Kolin, D.A.; Farley, K.X.; Wilson, J.M.; McLawhorn, A.S.; Cross, M.B.; Sculco, P.K. Projected economic burden of periprosthetic joint infection of the hip and knee in the united states. *J. Arthroplast.* **2021**, *36*, 1484–1489.e3. [CrossRef]
10. Parvizi, J.; Tan, T.L.; Goswami, K.; Higuera, C.; Della Valle, C.; Chen, A.F.; Shohat, N. The 2018 Definition of Periprosthetic Hip and Knee Infection: An Evidence-Based and Validated Criteria. *J. Arthroplast.* **2018**, *33*, 1309–1314.e2. [CrossRef]

11. Kheir, M.M.; Tan, T.L.; Ackerman, C.T.; Modi, R.; Foltz, C.; Parvizi, J. Culturing periprosthetic joint infection: Number of samples, growth duration, and organisms. *J. Arthroplast.* **2018**, *33*, 3531–3536.e1. [CrossRef] [PubMed]
12. Schäfer, P.; Fink, B.; Sandow, D.; Margull, A.; Berger, I.; Frommelt, L. Prolonged bacterial culture to identify late periprosthetic joint infection: A promising strategy. *Clin. Infect. Dis.* **2008**, *47*, 1403–1409. [CrossRef]
13. Talsma, D.T.; Ploegmakers, J.J.W.; Jutte, P.C.; Kampinga, G.; Wouthuyzen-Bakker, M. Time to positivity of acute and chronic periprosthetic joint infection cultures. *Diagn. Microbiol. Infect. Dis.* **2021**, *99*, 115178. [CrossRef]
14. Esteban, J.; Alvarez-Alvarez, B.; Blanco, A.; Fernández-Roblas, R.; Gadea, I.; Garcia-Cañete, J.; Sandoval, E.; Valdazo, M. Prolonged incubation time does not increase sensitivity for the diagnosis of implant-related infection using samples prepared by sonication of the implants. *Bone Jt. J.* **2013**, *95-B*, 1001–1006. [CrossRef]
15. Klement, M.R.; Cunningham, D.J.; Wooster, B.M.; Wellman, S.S.; Bolognesi, M.P.; Green, C.L.; Garrigues, G.E. Comparing standard versus extended culture duration in acute hip and knee periprosthetic joint infection. *J. Am. Acad. Orthop. Surg.* **2019**, *27*, e437–e443. [CrossRef] [PubMed]
16. Yusuf, E.; Roschka, C.; Esteban, J.; Raglio, A.; Tisler, A.; Willems, P.; Kramer, T.S. The State of Microbiology Diagnostic of Prosthetic Joint Infection in Europe: An In-Depth Survey Among Clinical Microbiologists. *Front. Microbiol.* **2022**, *13*, 906989. [CrossRef]
17. Osmon, D.R.; Berbari, E.F.; Berendt, A.R.; Lew, D.; Zimmerli, W.; Steckelberg, J.M.; Rao, N.; Hanssen, A.; Wilson, W.R. Diagnosis and Management of Prosthetic Joint Infection: Clinical Practice Guidelines by the Infectious Diseases Society of America. *Clin. Infect. Dis.* **2013**, *56*, e1–e25. [CrossRef]
18. American Academy of Orthopaedic Surgeons Evidence-Based Clinical Practice Guideline for Diagnosis and Prevention of Periprosthetic Joint Infections, AAOS. 2019. Available online: https://www.aaos.org/pjicpg (accessed on 14 February 2024).
19. von Elm, E.; Altman, D.G.; Egger, M.; Pocock, S.J.; Gøtzsche, P.C.; Vandenbroucke, J.P. STROBE Initiative the Strengthening the Reporting of Observational Studies in Epidemiology (STROBE) statement: Guidelines for reporting observational studies. *Ann. Intern. Med.* **2007**, *147*, 573–577. [CrossRef]
20. Fillingham, Y.A.; Della Valle, C.J.; Suleiman, L.I.; Springer, B.D.; Gehrke, T.; Bini, S.A.; Segreti, J.; Chen, A.F.; Goswami, K.; Tan, T.L.; et al. Definition of successful infection management and guidelines for reporting of outcomes after surgical treatment of periprosthetic joint infection: From the workgroup of the musculoskeletal infection society (MSIS). *J. Bone Jt. Surg. Am.* **2019**, *101*, e69. [CrossRef]
21. Coughlan, A.; Taylor, F. Classifications in brief: The McPherson classification of periprosthetic infection. *Clin. Orthop. Relat. Res.* **2020**, *478*, 903–908. [CrossRef]
22. Butler-Wu, S.M.; Burns, E.M.; Pottinger, P.S.; Magaret, A.S.; Rakeman, J.L.; Matsen, F.A.; Cookson, B.T. Optimization of periprosthetic culture for diagnosis of Propionibacterium acnes prosthetic joint infection. *J. Clin. Microbiol.* **2011**, *49*, 2490–2495. [CrossRef] [PubMed]
23. Renz, N.; Mudrovcic, S.; Perka, C.; Trampuz, A. Orthopedic implant-associated infections caused by *Cutibacterium* spp.—A remaining diagnostic challenge. *PLoS ONE* **2018**, *13*, e0202639. [CrossRef] [PubMed]
24. Hall, K.K.; Lyman, J.A. Updated review of blood culture contamination. *Clin. Microbiol. Rev.* **2006**, *19*, 788–802. [CrossRef]
25. Esposito, S.; Leone, S. Prosthetic joint infections: Microbiology, diagnosis, management and prevention. *Int. J. Antimicrob. Agents* **2008**, *32*, 287–293. [CrossRef] [PubMed]
26. Del Pozo, J.L.; Patel, R. Clinical practice. Infection associated with prosthetic joints. *N. Engl. J. Med.* **2009**, *361*, 787–794. [CrossRef]
27. Gupta, V.; Kaur, M.; Bora, P.; Kumari, P.; Datta, P.; Gupta, R.; Chander, J. A prospective study to assess the optimal incubation times for culture and aerobic bacterial profile in prosthetic joint infections. *J. Lab. Physicians* **2021**, *13*, 224–230. [CrossRef] [PubMed]
28. View of Risk of Treatment Failure for Prosthetic Joint Infections: Retrospective Chart Review in an Outpatient Parenteral Antimicrobial Therapy Program | Canadian *J. Hosp. Pharm.* **2023**, *76*, 1. Available online: https://www.cjhp-online.ca/index.php/cjhp/article/view/3264/4835 (accessed on 31 October 2023).
29. Kandel, C.E.; Jenkinson, R.; Daneman, N.; Backstein, D.; Hansen, B.E.; Muller, M.P.; Katz, K.C.; Widdifield, J.; Bogoch, E.; Ward, S.; et al. Predictors of Treatment Failure for Hip and Knee Prosthetic Joint Infections in the Setting of 1- and 2-Stage Exchange Arthroplasty: A Multicenter Retrospective Cohort. *Open Forum Infect. Dis.* **2019**, *6*, ofz452. [CrossRef]
30. Espíndola, R.; Vella, V.; Benito, N.; Mur, I.; Tedeschi, S.; Zamparini, E.; Hendriks, J.G.E.; Sorlí, L.; Murillo, O.; Soldevila, L.; et al. ARTHR-IS Group Rates and Predictors of Treatment Failure in Staphylococcus aureus Prosthetic Joint Infections According to Different Management Strategies: A Multinational Cohort Study-The ARTHR-IS Study Group. *Infect. Dis. Ther.* **2022**, *11*, 2177–2203. [CrossRef]
31. Flaten, D.; Berrigan, L.; Spirkina, A.; Gin, A. Risk of treatment failure for prosthetic joint infections: Retrospective chart review in an outpatient parenteral antimicrobial therapy program. *Can. J. Hosp. Pharm.* **2023**, *76*, 14–22. [CrossRef]
32. van Schaik, T.J.A.; de Jong, L.D.; van Meer, M.P.A.; Goosen, J.H.M.; Somford, M.P. The concordance between preoperative synovial fluid culture and intraoperative tissue cultures in periprosthetic joint infection: A systematic review. *J. Bone Jt. Infect.* **2022**, *7*, 259–267. [CrossRef]

33. Stone, W.Z.; Gray, C.F.; Parvataneni, H.K.; Al-Rashid, M.; Vlasak, R.G.; Horodyski, M.; Prieto, H.A. Clinical Evaluation of Synovial Alpha Defensin and Synovial C-Reactive Protein in the Diagnosis of Periprosthetic Joint Infection. *J. Bone Jt. Surg. Am.* **2018**, *100*, 1184–1190. [CrossRef]
34. Stone, W.Z.; Gray, C.F.; Parvataneni, H.K.; Prieto, H.A. Clinical evaluation of alpha defensin test following staged treatment of prosthetic joint infections. *J. Arthroplasty* **2019**, *34*, 1446–1451. [CrossRef]

Disclaimer/Publisher's Note: The statements, opinions and data contained in all publications are solely those of the individual author(s) and contributor(s) and not of MDPI and/or the editor(s). MDPI and/or the editor(s) disclaim responsibility for any injury to people or property resulting from any ideas, methods, instructions or products referred to in the content.

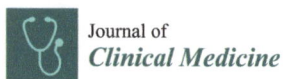

Article

Functional Outcome after Direct Anterior Approach Total Hip Arthroplasty (DAA-THA) for Coxa Profunda and Protrusio Acetabuli—A Retrospective Study

Tizian Heinz [1], Hristo Vasilev [1], Philip Mark Anderson [1], Ioannis Stratos [1], Axel Jakuscheit [1], Konstantin Horas [1], Boris Michael Holzapfel [2], Maximilian Rudert [1] and Manuel Weißenberger [1,*]

[1] Department of Orthopaedic Surgery, University of Wuerzburg, Koenig-Ludwig-Haus, Brettreichstr 11, 97074 Wuerzburg, Germany; t-heinz.klh@uni-wuerzburg.de (T.H.); hrs.vasilev@gmail.com (H.V.); p-anderson.klh@uni-wuerzburg.de (P.M.A.); i-stratos.klh@uni-wuerzburg.de (I.S.); a-jakuscheit.klh@uni-wuerzburg.de (A.J.); k-horas.klh@uni-wuerzburg.de (K.H.); m-rudert.klh@uni-wuerzburg.de (M.R.)
[2] Department of Orthopedics and Trauma Surgery, Musculoskeletal University Center, Munich (MUM), University Hospital, LMU Munich, Marchioninistr 15, 81377 Munich, Germany; boris.holzapfel@med.uni-muenchen.de
* Correspondence: manuel.weissenberger@googlemail.com

Abstract: **Objective:** The direct anterior approach (DAA) is a recognized technique for total hip arthroplasty (THA) that spares soft tissue. Functional and clinical outcomes following THA via the DAA in patients with complex acetabular deformities, specifically coxa profunda (CP) and protrusio acetabuli (PA), have yet to be determined. **Methods:** A retrospective analysis was conducted on 188 primary THA cases, including 100 CP hips and 88 PA hips, performed via the DAA. Functional and clinical outcomes were evaluated by means of the Western Ontario and McMaster Universities Arthritis Index (WOMAC) and Harris Hip Score (HHS) preoperatively and at a mean follow-up of 46 ± 14 months. Furthermore, potential complications were assessed. **Results:** From the preoperative to the latest postoperative visit, a significant improvement in the WOMAC total score was observed (CP: −34.89 ± 20.66; PA: −40.38 ± 21.11). The length of stay (LOS) was the only parameter predictive of the postoperative WOMAC total score, with each day of LOS increasing the postoperative WOMAC by a mean of 1.77 points ($p < 0.01$). The HHS improved by 38.37 ± 14.23 (PA-group) and 32.79 ± 14.89 points (CP-group). No significant difference in the patient-reported outcome measures (PROMs) between the CP- and PA-group was found. The survival rate for any revision was 97.70% (PA-group) and 92.80% (CP-group). **Conclusion:** The results of this study indicate that the minimally invasive DAA was not predictive of the functional and clinical outcome following DAA-THA in patients with CP and PA. Improvements in the mean WOMAC and HHS scores were above or within the reported MCID. Additionally, revision rates were well below those reported in the literature for short and intermediate follow-up periods.

Keywords: total hip arthroplasty; direct anterior approach (DAA); coxa profunda; protrusio acetabuli

1. Introduction

Total hip arthroplasty (THA) has become the preferred treatment for symptomatic and advanced osteoarthritis (OA) of the hip joint, alleviating pain and restoring pain-free joint function. Due to its high success rate, THA is often referred to as the surgery of the century [1].

Despite the highly standardized surgical procedure, anatomical abnormalities such as dysplasia, coxa profunda (CP), and protrusio acetabuli (PA) pose significant challenges to the surgeon and may hamper the postoperative outcome if not adequately addressed prior to surgery. CP describes an extensively deep socket, with the floor of the acetabula fossa medial to the ilioischial line on a.p. hip radiographs [2]. In contrast, the more severe form, protrusio acetabuli (PA), is defined by medialization or protrusion of the femoral head into the acetabular fossa which can be seen on a.p. hip radiographs as the medial aspect of the femoral head lying medial to the ilioischial line [2–4]. Thus, PA is associated with a defect or insufficiency of the medial acetabular wall, allowing for the medial protrusion of the femoral head into the acetabular fossa and lesser pelvis. The deficient medial wall and compromised bone of the acetabular rim may yield significant intraoperative challenges that need to be anticipated during the templating and planning process prior to surgery [5–7]. In addition, CP and PA are often associated with a varus neck-shaft angle, which often leads to incarceration of the femoral head into the acetabular fossa, rendering femoral neck osteotomy during arthroplasty rather difficult [8]. Whilst the underlying causes of CP and PA are mostly unknown, up to 5% are reported to develop secondary to rheumatoid arthritis [6,7]. However, the prevalence of CP and PA in the general population is widely unexplored and thought to be less than 1% [9]. Some authors suggest a female predominance [10,11].

THA is the preferred treatment option for patients with CP or PA and advanced symptomatic OA of the hip joint. However, reconstruction of the native hip biomechanics warrants special attention in CP and PA because of the associated medialization and proximalization of the hip joint center. Various techniques have been reported for addressing the medial defect of the acetabular wall, with procedures including acetabuloplasty with morselized allograft or autograft harvested from the resected femoral head in conjunction with cemented and cementless cups [12–15]. However, the usage of bone cement alone or in conjunction with bone graft has been reported to have unsatisfactory results due to early migration and loosening of the implanted cups [12,14–16]. Promising results in managing THA in patients with PA have recently been reported with cementless cups, with additional autologous bone grafting if needed [8,15,17,18]. However, none of the aforementioned studies have investigated the feasibility and suitability of the minimal invasive direct anterior approach (DAA) in the treatment of PA and CP.

Serving as the rationale of this retrospective study, the results and the potential influential factors associated with cementless cup THA in conjunction with the aspiring minimal invasive DAA for PA and CP were yet to be investigated [18,19]. It was hypothesized that the minimally invasive nature of the DAA would not be adversely associated with the typically observed performance of cementless cups in PA and CP cases.

2. Materials and Methods

This cohort study was organized and reported in accordance with the STROBE (strengthening the reporting of observational studies in epidemiology, www.strobe-statement.org) checklist, ensuring a clear presentation of the conducted observational study [20].

2.1. Study Population

A cohort study design was used, and by retrospective medical record review at a single university center for orthopedic surgery in Germany, a total of 188 patients were found to be eligible for the study, as reported previously [18]. Medical records were reviewed for eligibility between September 2017 and February 2020. The inclusion criteria were based on established clinical and radiographic findings advocating and justifying the THA procedure: (1) radiographic confirmation of severe hip osteoarthritis, at least Kellgren–Lawrence grade III [21], and (2) hip osteoarthritis-contingent symptoms with ongoing pain, compromised joint function, and reduced walking distance [21,22]. Specifically, as per the primary intention of this study, the (3) inclusion of the DAA as the only surgical approach for THA was mandatory, as well as (4) radiographic evidence of CP or PA. After radiographic review, 88 and 100 patients were assigned to the PA-group and CP-group, respectively. Clinical outcomes were assessed using established patient reported outcome measurers (PROMs) that were routinely evaluated at specific time points related to the arthroplasty procedure (Table 1). However, only patients with a complete set of pre- and postoperatively available PROMs were evaluated, accounting for 23 and 16 patients in the PA- and CP-group, respectively (Figure 1). PROMs were defined as the primary outcome parameter. The severity of medial acetabular wall insufficiency (CP or in more severe cases PA) was thought to be a predictor of the surgical outcome parameters. In an attempt to reduce potential bias, clearly defined inclusion and exclusion criteria were used throughout the study. Furthermore, standardized forms and procedures for data collection were used to ensure consistency and systematic evaluation of potentially relevant parameters, thereby reducing the risk of confounding variables. Recall bias was addressed by reporting only on evaluated and well-established PROMs. Inclusion and exclusion criteria were not modified during the study, thereby addressing selection bias. Surgical complications and all readmissions related to the index procedure were evaluated. Mean follow-up was 3.84 years. This study was submitted to and approved by the local Ethics Committee (Nr. 20200619 01), ensuring accordance with the Declaration of Helsinki [23].

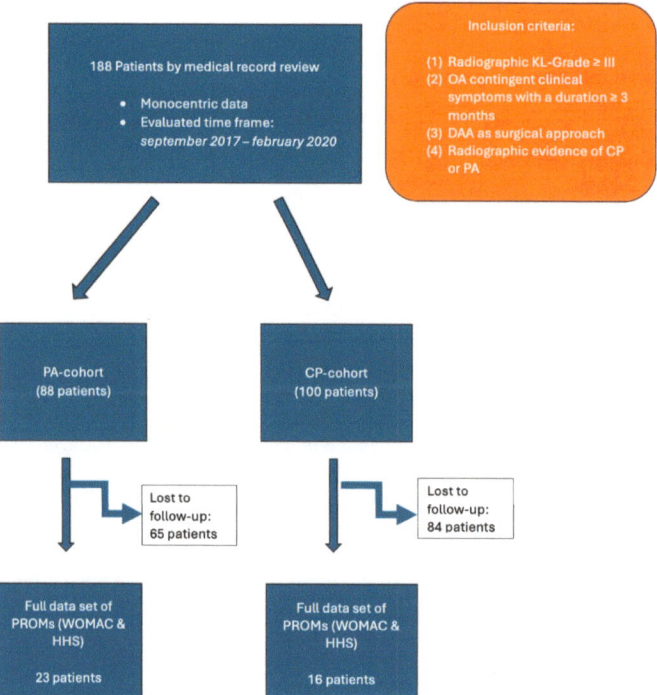

Figure 1. Summarizing the study design.

Table 1. Type and timing of PROMs during the study period.

Type of PROM	Time of Evaluation
EQ5D	Preoperative
	1 year postoperative
	5 years postoperative
WOMAC	Preoperative
	1 year postoperative
	5 years postoperative
Harris Hip Score (HHS)	Preoperative
	3 years postoperative
VAS	Preoperative
	1 year postoperative

2.2. Surgical Technique

This study used the widely practiced surgical approach known as the direct anterior approach (DAA) [18,19]. To outline the procedure, patients were positioned supine on a standard operating table, and landmarks such as the greater trochanter (GT) and the anterior superior iliac spine (ASIS) were marked out prior to incision. Approximately 3 cm distal and lateral to the ASIS, the starting point for the incision could be found [24]. The incision was then extended about 5 to 6 cm distally in the direction of the lateral distal femoral condyle and the head of the fibula. Then, the fascia overlying the tensor fasciae latae (TFL) was exposed and dissected along its fibers, revealing the Hueter interval between the sartorius muscle and the TFL [24]. Subsequently, the branches of the lateral circumflex femoral vessels were ligated, followed by the femoral neck osteotomy for removal of the femoral head. Abductor tenotomy was commonly avoided by obtaining deep muscle relaxation under general anesthesia prior to head removal. Autologous morselized bone chips from the resected femoral head were utilized for augmentation in cases of extensive medial wall defects [7]. The cup was cemented in cases where there was limited stability or severe osteoporosis. After placement of the cup and liner, insertion of a bone hook into the proximal femoral canal while bringing the limb in hyperextension, adduction, and external rotation gave sufficient access for subsequent broaching. Visualization of the femoral canal was additionally improved by releasing the posterior capsule and placing a Mueller retractor under the GT [24]. The femoral canal was broached until a press fit and rotational stability was reached. The hip joint was then tested with the trial implant. Once adequate joint stability and acceptable leg length discrepancy (LLD) were achieved, the trial implant was replaced with the permanent implant of the same size, followed by intraoperative fluoroscopic verification [24]. Prior to wound closure, 2 g of tranexamic acid was injected into the hip joint. All procedures were performed by seven senior surgeons (J.A., B.H., S.B., M.R., R.S., M.W., and M.L.) using identical sets of surgical instruments. Zimmer Biomet's ML-Taper femoral prosthesis and Allofit S Alloclassic acetabular cup were used consistently throughout the procedures.

2.3. Radiographic Features

Pelvic radiographs were taken using a standardized procedure and meticulously checked for tilt or rotation discrepancies before templating and measurement. These images were digitally archived using the Picture Archiving and Communication System (PACS), and measurements were performed using the angle and measurement tools available in the X-ray viewer (DeepUnity Review, DH Healthcare GmbH, Bonn, Germany). All measurements were performed on plain standing anteroposterior pelvic radiographs with 15 degrees of internal rotation [2].

Radiomorphologic features were used to differentiate between CP and PA: CP was identified when the medial wall of the acetabular fossa was medial to the ilioischial line while the medial cortex of the femoral head remained lateral or aligned with the ilioischial line. Conversely, PA was identified when both the medial wall of the acetabular fossa and the medial cortex of the femoral head were medial to the ilioischial line. In addition, the degree of PA was further delineated by measuring the horizontal distance between the ilioischial line (also referred to as the Kohler line) and the medial acetabular margin, referred to as the AK distance. After surgery, the medial edge of the acetabular component served as a substitute for the medial acetabular wall. Based on the AK distance, gradations were established: (1) 1 to 5 mm was indicative of mild PA, (2) 6 to 15 mm was indicative of moderate PA, and (3) AK distance greater than 16 mm was indicative of severe PA [19]. A detailed radiographic analysis of this patient cohort has been described elsewhere [18].

2.4. Statistical Analysis

Data analysis was conducted using SPSS software (version 27, SPSS Inc., Chicago, IL, USA). Ordinal variables were presented as means with standard deviations, while categorical variables were described using absolute and relative frequencies. The Kolmogorov–

Smirnov test was employed to assess the normality of data distribution. Group differences between CP and PA were analyzed using either the independent *t*-test or the Mann–Whitney U test. Categorical variable frequencies were compared using the chi-square test. Within-group differences over time (preoperative to postoperative) were evaluated using the dependent *t*-test or Wilcoxon test. Additionally, logistic and linear regression analyses were performed to investigate the impact of several independent factors on the outcome variables, thereby adjusting for confounding variables. A priori sample size calculation was performed using G-power (version 3.1) [25], assuming a conservative effect size and a statistical power of 0.8, which translated to a total sample size of 38 patients. A significance threshold was set at $p < 0.05$.

3. Results

3.1. Patient Demographics

A total of 188 patients were included in the study cohort, with 88 and 100 patients being assigned to the PA-group and CP-group, respectively. A strong predominance of female patients was found in both cohorts. The mean age was significantly higher in the PA-group compared to patients with coxa profunda. A significant correlation was found between hip morphology (protrusio acetabuli and coxa profunda) and the type of THA fixation, with CP patients having a higher likelihood of cementless fixation ($p = 0.01$). Patient demographics and characteristics are shown in Table 2.

Table 2. Patient demographics and characteristics.

Item	PA-Group	CP-Group	
	Mean (±SD), rel. frequency		*p*-value (CP-group vs. PA-group)
Age (years ± SD)	71.61 ± 12.41	67.05 ± 10.23	0.01
ASA	I: 1 (1.1%) II: 56 (63.6%) III: 30 (34.1%) IV: 1 (1.1%)	I: 6 (6.0%) II: 65 (65.0%) III: 28 (28.0%) IV: 1 (1.0%)	0.31
BMI (kg/m^2)	27.24 ± 4.61	27.91 ± 5.25	0.36
Sex (female/male)	75/13, 85.20%/14.80%	82/18, 82.0%/18.0%	0.35
Hip flexion preoperative (degrees)	82.63 ± 17.80	90.20 ± 16.60	0.00
Hip flexion postoperative (degrees)	112.14 ± 9.17	101.67 ± 20.05	0.02
Method of fixation (cementless/hybrid/fully cemented)	72/11/5	94/6/0	0.01
LOS (days ± SD)	9.11 ± 3.58	8.44 ± 2.10	0.11

3.2. Radiographic Outcome

When stratified according to the AK distance, 33 and 50 patients were identified with mild and moderate PA. Moreover, five cases with severe PA defined by an AK distance greater than 16 mm were found. Postoperatively, the PA was fully treated in 59 cases (67.05%) by transferring the medial border of the acetabular component lateral to or flush with the ilioischial line. In the remaining 29 cases, the PA was not fully treated, but the AK distance was reduced by a mean of 3.93 ± 4.53 mm. A more detailed radiographic analysis of this study cohort has been previously reported [18].

3.3. Clinical Outcome and PROMs

A significant decrease in the WOMAC total score and WOMAC subscores were observed in both the CP- and PA-groups from the preoperative to the postoperative visit (Figure 2). The mean improvement for the CP- and PA-groups at the last follow-up visit was −34.89 ± 20.66 and −40.38 ± 21.11, respectively (Table 3). Prior to surgery, there were no statistically significant differences in the WOMAC total score or its subscores between the CP- and PA-groups. The observed improvement was similar across both groups, with no statistically significant differences in WOMAC total and subscores at the last follow-up (Table 3). The length of stay (LOS) was the only parameter predictive for the postoperative

WOMAC total score, with every day of LOS increasing the postoperative WOMAC by a mean of 1.77 points ($p < 0.01$).

Regarding the HHS, patients with PA had a lower mean HHS compared to patients with CP at the preoperative visit, though it was not statistically significant (Figure 3). Both the CP- and PA-group showed a significant improvement from the preoperative to the postoperative visit ($p < 0.01$), with mean improvements in the HHS of 38.37 ± 14.23 (PA-group) and 32.79 ± 14.89 (CP-group), respectively. At the last follow-up, values of the HHS were not statistically different between the CP- and PA-group.

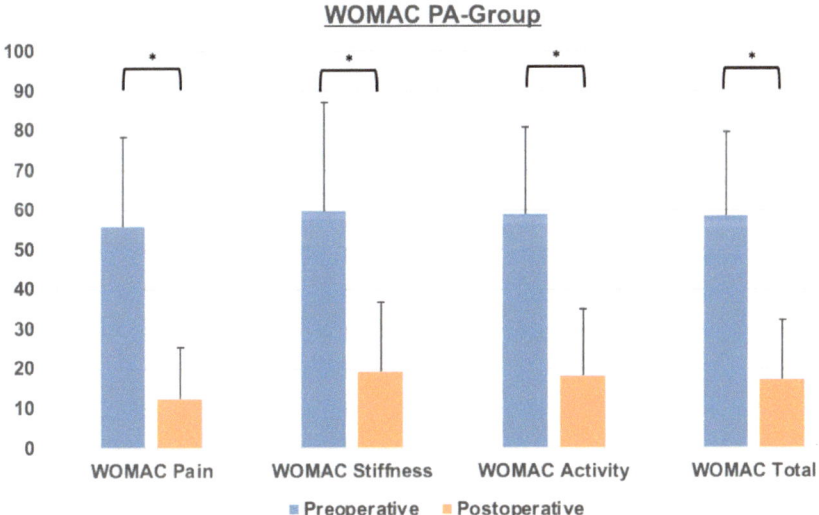

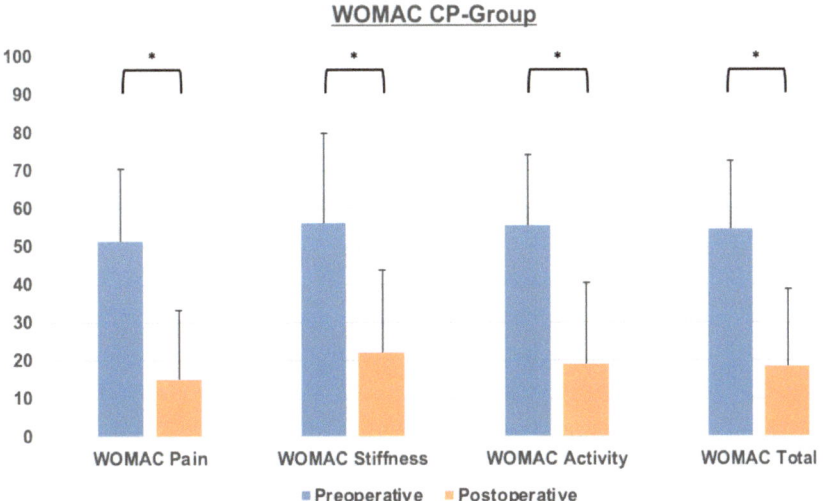

Figure 2. Pre- and postoperative WOMAC scores for the PA- and CP-groups. Significant differences ($p < 0.05$) are marked by asterisks.

The LOS, ASA, and change in hemoglobin (Delta HB) were the only parameters showing a significant correlative association with postoperative HHS.

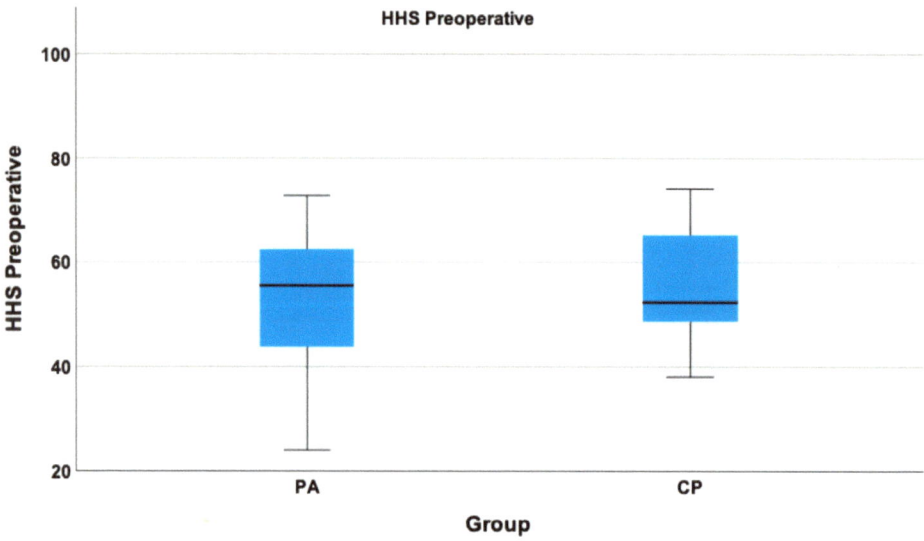

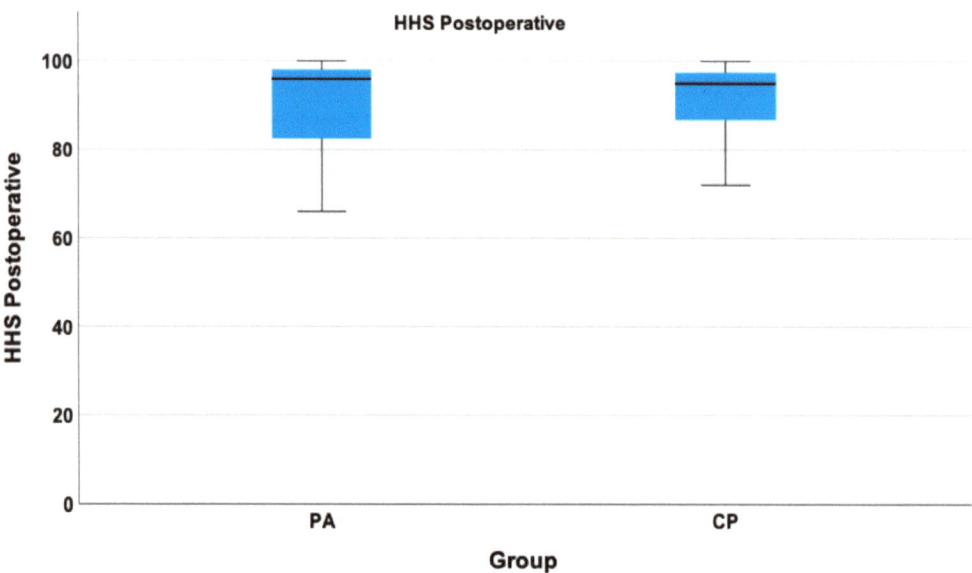

Figure 3. Pre- and postoperative HHS scores for the CP- and PA-group.

Table 3. Pre- and postoperative WOMAC scores for the CP- and PA-group. Significances for within-group changes and between-group changes are given.

	CP-Group	PA-Group	p-Value (CP-Group vs. PA-Group)
WOMAC Pain preoperative	51.60 ± 19.00	55.86 + 22.39	0.17
WOMAC Pain postoperative	15.08 ± 18.06	12.60 ± 12.79	0.36
p-value (preoperative vs. postoperative)	<0.00	<0.00	
WOMAC Stiffness preoperative	56.16 ± 23.83	59.73 ± 19.21	0.35
WOMAC Stiffness postoperative	22.10 ± 21.70	19.21 ± 17.51	0.39
p-value (preoperative vs. postoperative)	<0.00	<0.00	
WOMAC Activity preoperative	55.61 ± 18.45	58.94 ± 18.12	0.26
WOMAC Activity postoperative	19.18 ± 21.30	18.16 ± 16.81	0.76
p-value (preoperative vs. postoperative)	<0.00	<0.00	
WOMAC Total preoperative	54.65 ± 17.83	58.52 ± 20.94	0.18
WOMAC Total postoperative	18.58 ± 20.11	17.15 ± 15.07	0.64
p-value (preoperative vs. postoperative)	<0.00	<0.00	

Furthermore, there was a statistically significant linear association of the BMI and the duration of surgery, with every increase in the BMI by one unit leading to an elevated surgery time of 0.91 min ($R^2 = 0.06$, $F(1) = 12.57$, $p = 0.01$) (Figure 4). However, duration of surgery was not significantly different in both groups, with a mean OR-time of 59.10 ± 17.75 min.

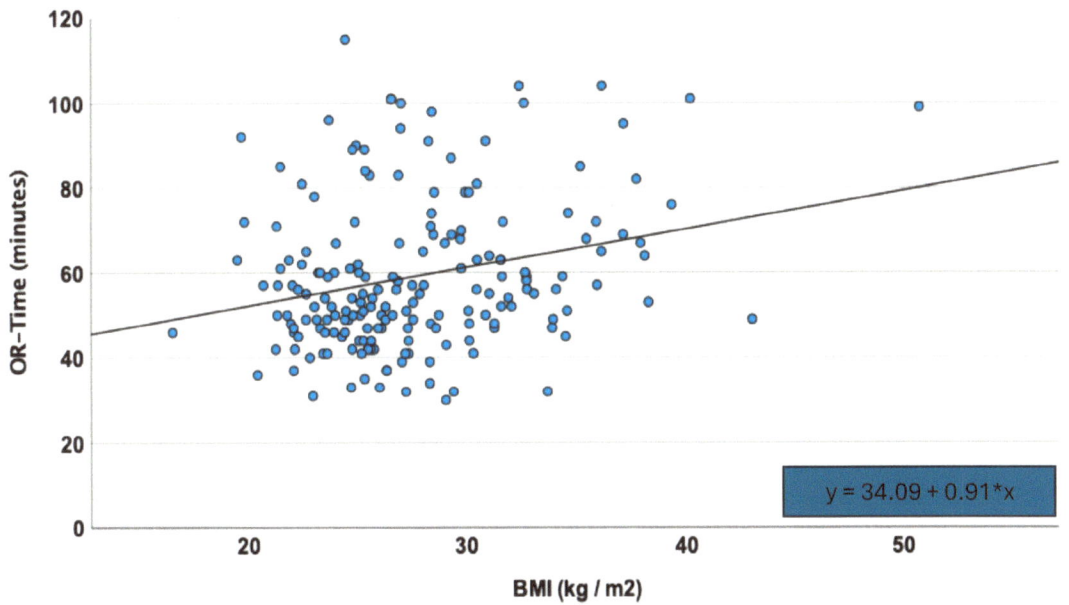

Figure 4. Correlative association of the BMI and the OR-time by linear regression analysis.

The mean hemoglobin drop from the preoperative to the postoperative visit (3 days after surgery) turned out to be 2.79 ± 1.14 g/dL, without any significant difference in both groups.

Intraoperative and postoperative complications, such as anemia, respiratory infection, prolonged wound healing, or nerve injury, showed no significant differences between the two groups (Table 4). In the PA-group, two patients required revision surgery at 3 and 4 weeks postoperatively due to acetabular cup loosening (one case) and superficial wound infection (one case). In the CP-group, one patient underwent revision of the femoral component 4 weeks postoperatively due to a periprosthetic fracture. Additionally, two patients in the CP-group were readmitted at 8 weeks and another patient at 2 years, all due to periprosthetic infection. The mean follow-up period screened for readmission at the index hospital was 50.13 months. Survival analysis showed no significant difference for the PA- and CP-group, with a survival rate of 97.70% and 92.80% during the mean follow-up period for the PA- and CP-group for any revision as endpoint. With acetabular loosening as the endpoint, the survival rate in the CP-group and PA-group was 100% and 98.90%, respectively.

Table 4. Complication rates of the CP- and PA-group during the follow-up period of a mean of 50.13 months.

	CP-Group	PA-Group
Complication rates (total number n, percent %)		
Postoperative anemia	3 (3.00%)	2 (2.27%)
Prolonged wound healing	4 (4.00%)	4 (4.54%)
Postoperative regional paresthesia	2 (2.00%)	1 (1.14%)
Respiratory infection	2 (2.00%)	2 (2.27%)
Intraoperative fracture (femur or acetabulum)	1 (0.53%)	2 (1.06%)

4. Discussion

PA and CP, though relatively rare, represent a complex hip morphology, rendering primary hip arthroplasty a complex surgical procedure. It was the primary intention of this study to investigate whether complex hip deformities such as CP and PA are still associated with favorable PROMs when undergoing arthroplasty through the minimally invasive DAA. With the recent extension of the DAA to hip revision cases, it was hypothesized that complex primary hip deformities like CP and PA would not be influenced by the minimally invasive nature of the DAA. Furthermore, the authors have recently demonstrated promising radiographic results following primary THA in CP and PA cases [18], but the relation with clinical outcome data was still lacking.

As a main finding of this study, cementless cup THA performed through the minimally invasive DAA was associated with satisfying and promising patient-reported outcome measures in the cases of both PA and CP. Specifically, in the CP-group and PA-group, the mean increase in the HHS from preoperative to the last visit turned out to be 32.79 ± 14.89 and 38.37 ± 14.23 points. Singh et al. reported a minimal clinically important difference (MCID) for the HHS of 18.0 and 15.9 points following two and five years from the arthroplasty procedure [26]. With the HHS change score of this study cohort being significantly higher than the reported MCID, a clinically important gain in function and pain was inferred. Similarly, the mean change score for WOMAC Pain turned out to be well within the reported MCID for both groups [27]. Regarding the WOMAC Function subscore, the mean change scores (CP: 35.18 ± 21.86; PA: 40.12 ± 21.30) were well within the reported MCID [27]. Therefore, based on the results of the HHS and WOMAC scores, a remarkably high gain in function and pain was observed in both groups after hip arthroplasty with the DAA.

Traditionally, cementation of the acetabular component for the management of PA has been suggested for a while. The idea behind this outdated recommendation was that the bone cement would aid in supporting and bridging the deficient medial wall and facilitate placement of the cup in a more anatomical position [14,17,28,29]. However, the mid- and long-term data showed a remarkably high rate of aseptic acetabular loosening and recurrence of acetabular protrusion in those cases treated with cementation of the acetabular component, leading to a paradigm shift towards the use of cementless cups with or without autologous bone support, demonstrating promising results [7,30,31]. Similarly, Baghdadi et al. demonstrated a considerably higher mid- and long-term survival rate of the socket when using a non-cemented porous coated cup compared to a cemented cup [8,32]. Regardless of the fixation technique, meticulous reconstruction of the center of the native rotation (COR), which is usually moved superiorly and medially due to the medial acetabular defect, has been identified as a major predictor determining the survival rate of the acetabular component. Thus, a 24% risk of aseptic cup loosening has been associated with each 1 mm of undercorrection of the native COR [32,33]. Reported survival rates of the implant following THA range from 80% to 90% for short and intermediate follow-up periods [33–35]. With a survival rate of 97.8% in this study cohort, a slightly better mean survival for any surgical revision than what is commonly reported in the literature was found. This finding is also supported by the satisfying and promising radiographic reconstruction parameters achieved in this study cohort [18].

Another noteworthy finding of this study was that the clinical outcome data between the CP- and PA-group did not have a statistically significant difference. Since CP is generally considered a less complicated anatomical variant compared to PA, this finding suggests that the surgical approach to the hip joint may not significantly influence the outcomes of complex hip arthroplasty.

To the knowledge of the authors, this is the first study reporting on the DAA for the management of CP and PA on a large patient cohort. Recently, the DAA has experienced an unprecedented rise worldwide due to its minimally invasive and tissue-sparing nature [36]. This has led to a gradual expansion of the DAA to more complex primary THA cases such as developmental dysplasia of the hip (DDH), and revision arthroplasty via the DAA has also recently been reported [37,38]. The main idea behind this trend is to transfer the potential merits of the DAA to complex primary THA, namely early postoperative mobilization, less intraoperative blood loss, and decreased dislocation risk [39,40].

In conclusion, the DAA seems to not constitute a limiting factor in the management of OA in patients with medial acetabular protrusion. The large increase in common PROMs demonstrates a significant gain in hip function and decrease in hip pain in the study cohort. This sharp improvement of the WOMAC and HHS scores during the follow-up period may be partially due to the minimally invasive nature of the DAA. Meanwhile, several studies have exhibited a significant benefit of the DAA at the short and intermediate follow-up [40–42]. Furthermore, the uncomplicated implementation of fluoroscopy in conjunction with the DAA facilitates intraoperative control of cup placement and eases restoring of the COR.

It is noteworthy, given the retrospective nature of this study, that there are inevitably some shortcomings: firstly, the lack of a control group limits the generalizability of the results from this study cohort. Secondly, an extension of the follow-up period to at least ten years would have aided in examining the long-term fate and revision rates of the DAA-THA. Notably, there was a strong predominance of female patients, which may cause potential bias. However, CP and PA are known to have a strong female predominance, and multi-variate regression analysis did not find gender to be a potentially confounding variable.

This study is, to our knowledge, the first to explore the clinical outcome of the DAA for complex THA in CP and PA patients. The substantial sample size of 100 hips in the PA-group increases the robustness of the results. Therefore, the findings of the present study may serve as a starting point for future research on this topic, and prospective study designs will be needed to finally evaluate the safety and efficacy of the DAA in conjunction with complex PA and CP hip arthroplasty.

5. Conclusions

The results of this study indicate that the minimally invasive DAA was not predictive of the functional and clinical outcome following DAA-THA in patients with CP and PA. Improvements in the mean WOMAC and HHS scores were above or within the reported MCID. Additionally, revision rates were well below those reported in the literature for short and intermediate follow-up periods.

Author Contributions: All authors contributed equally to the manuscript. T.H. and M.W. were involved in the study design and manuscript drafting. H.V. and I.S. were responsible for data acquisition and interpretation. The data analysis was performed by T.H., P.M.A. and A.J. B.M.H. and M.R. were responsible for study supervision and were major contributors to writing the manuscript. M.R., M.W. and K.H. were involved in data interpretation and designing the study. All authors have read and agreed to the published version of the manuscript.

Funding: The APC of this publication was funded by the Open Access Publication Fund of the University of Wuerzburg.

Institutional Review Board Statement: This study was conducted in accordance with the Declaration of Helsinki and approved by the Institutional Review Board of the University of Wuerzburg on 20 August 2020 (20200619 01).

Informed Consent Statement: Informed and written consent was obtained from all subjects involved in the study.

Data Availability Statement: Data can be obtained from the authors upon reasonable request.

Conflicts of Interest: The authors declare no conflicts of interest.

References

1. Learmonth, I.D.; Young, C.; Rorabeck, C. The operation of the century: Total hip replacement. *Lancet* **2007**, *370*, 1508–1519. [CrossRef] [PubMed]
2. Clohisy, J.C.; Carlisle, J.C.; Beaulé, P.E.; Kim, Y.J.; Trousdale, R.T.; Sierra, R.J.; Leunig, M.; Schoenecker, P.L.; Millis, M.B. A systematic approach to the plain radiographic evaluation of the young adult hip. *J. Bone Jt. Surg. Am.* **2008**, *90* (Suppl. 4), 47–66. [CrossRef] [PubMed]
3. Armbuster, T.G.; Guerra, J., Jr.; Resnick, D.; Goergen, T.G.; Feingold, M.L.; Niwayama, G.; Danzig, L.A. The adult hip: An anatomic study. Part I: The bony landmarks. *Radiology* **1978**, *128*, 1–10. [CrossRef] [PubMed]
4. Guerra, J., Jr.; Armbuster, T.G.; Resnick, D.; Goergen, T.G.; Feingold, M.L.; Niwayama, G.; Danzig, L.A. The adult hip: An anatomic study. Part II: The soft-tissue landmarks. *Radiology* **1978**, *128*, 11–20. [CrossRef] [PubMed]
5. Liu, P.; Qiao, Y.-J.; Lou, J.-P.; Cao, G.; Chang, Y.; Zhou, S.-H. Cementless total hip arthroplasty for treatment of acetabular protrusion secondary to rheumatoid arthritis. *J. Orthop. Surg. Res.* **2023**, *18*, 282. [CrossRef] [PubMed]
6. Lu, N.; Yang, Y.; Chen, H.; Li, W.; Pu, B.; Liu, L. Health-type total hip arthroplasty combined with compression bone grafting for rheumatoid arthritis with acetabular retraction. *Chin. J. Reconstr. Surg.* **2015**, *29*, 160–162.
7. Zhen, P.; Li, X.; Zhou, S.; Lu, H.; Chen, H.; Liu, J. Total hip arthroplasty to treat acetabular protrusions secondary to rheumatoid arthritis. *J. Orthop. Surg. Res.* **2018**, *13*, 92. [CrossRef]
8. Baghdadi, Y.M.K.; Larson, A.N.; Sierra, R.J. Long-term results of the uncemented acetabular component in a primary total hip arthroplasty performed for protrusio acetabuli: A fifteen year median follow-up. *Int. Orthop.* **2015**, *39*, 839–845. [CrossRef] [PubMed]
9. McBride, M.T.; Muldoon, M.P.; Santore, R.F.; Trousdale, R.T.; Wenger, D.R. Protrusio acetabuli: Diagnosis and treatment. *J. Am. Acad. Orthop. Surg.* **2001**, *9*, 79–88. [CrossRef]
10. Gilmour, J. Adolescent deformities of the acetabulum: An investigation into the nature of protrusio acetabuli. *Br. J. Surg.* **2005**, *26*, 670–699. [CrossRef]
11. Alexander, C. The Aetiology of Primary Protrusio Acetabuli. *Br. J. Radiol.* **1965**, *38*, 567–580. [CrossRef]
12. Hirst, P.; Esser, M.; Murphy, J.C.; Hardinge, K. Bone grafting for protrusio acetabuli during total hip replacement. A review of the Wrightington method in 61 hips. *J. Bone Jt. Surg. Br.* **1987**, *69*, 229–233. [CrossRef]
13. Garcia-Cimbrelo, E.; Diaz-Martin, A.; Madero, R.; Munera, L. Loosening of the cup after low-friction arthroplasty in patients with acetabular protrusion. The importance of the position of the cup. *J. Bone Jt. Surg. Br.* **2000**, *82*, 108–115. [CrossRef]
14. Welten, M.L.; Schreurs, B.W.; Buma, P.; Verdonschot, N.; Slooff, T.J. Acetabular reconstruction with impacted morcellized cancellous bone autograft and cemented primary total hip arthroplasty: A 10- to 17-year follow-up study. *J. Arthroplast.* **2000**, *15*, 819–824. [CrossRef]
15. Mullaji, A.B.; Shetty, G.M. Acetabular protrusio: Surgical technique of dealing with a problem in depth. *Bone Jt. J.* **2013**, *95-b* (Suppl. A), 37–40. [CrossRef]
16. Zuh, S.-G.; Zazgyva, A.; Gergely, I.; Pop, T.S. Acetabuloplasty with bone grafting in uncemented hip replacement for protrusion. *Int. Orthop.* **2015**, *39*, 1757–1763. [CrossRef] [PubMed]
17. Mullaji, A.B.; Marawar, S.V. Primary total hip arthroplasty in protrusio acetabuli using impacted morsellized bone grafting and cementless cups: A medium-term radiographic review. *J. Arthroplast.* **2007**, *22*, 1143–1149. [CrossRef] [PubMed]
18. Heinz, T.; Vasilev, H.; Anderson, P.M.; Stratos, I.; Jakuscheit, A.; Horas, K.; Holzapfel, B.M.; Rudert, M.; Weißenberger, M. The Direct Anterior Approach (DAA) as a Standard Approach for Total Hip Arthroplasty (THA) in Coxa Profunda and Protrusio Acetabuli? A Radiographic Analysis of 188 Cases. *J. Clin. Med.* **2023**, *12*, 3941. [CrossRef]

19. Yun, A.; Qutami, M.; Carles, E. Managing Protrusio Acetabuli With a Direct Anterior Approach Total Hip Replacement. *Cureus* **2021**, *13*, e14048. [CrossRef]
20. Cuschieri, S. The STROBE guidelines. *Saudi J. Anaesth.* **2019**, *13* (Suppl. 1), S31–S34. [CrossRef]
21. Günther, K.P.; Deckert, S.; Lützner, C.; Lange, T.; Schmitt, J.; Postler, A. Total Hip Replacement for Osteoarthritis-Evidence-Based and Patient-Oriented Indications. *Dtsch. Arztebl. Int.* **2021**, *118*, 730–736. [CrossRef]
22. Lützner, C.; Deckert, S.; Günther, K.-P.; Postler, A.E.; Lützner, J.; Schmitt, J.; Limb, D.; Lange, T. Indication Criteria for Total Hip Arthroplasty in Patients with Hip Osteoarthritis—Recommendations from a German Consensus Initiative. *Medicina* **2022**, *58*, 574. [CrossRef] [PubMed]
23. Association, W.M. World Medical Association Declaration of Helsinki: Ethical Principles for Medical Research Involving Human Subjects. *JAMA* **2013**, *310*, 2191–2194. [CrossRef]
24. Rudert, M.; Thaler, M.; Holzapfel, B.M. Primary hip arthroplasty via the direct anterior approach. *Oper. Orthop. Traumatol.* **2021**, *33*, 287. [CrossRef]
25. Faul, F.; Erdfelder, E.; Lang, A.G.; Buchner, A. G*Power 3: A flexible statistical power analysis program for the social, behavioral, and biomedical sciences. *Behav. Res. Methods* **2007**, *39*, 175–191. [CrossRef] [PubMed]
26. Singh, J.A.; Schleck, C.; Harmsen, S.; Lewallen, D. Clinically important improvement thresholds for Harris Hip Score and its ability to predict revision risk after primary total hip arthroplasty. *BMC Musculoskelet. Disord.* **2016**, *17*, 256. [CrossRef] [PubMed]
27. MacKay, C.; Clements, N.; Wong, R.; Davis, A.M. A systematic review of estimates of the minimal clinically important difference and patient acceptable symptom state of the Western Ontario and McMaster Universities Osteoarthritis Index in patients who underwent total hip and total knee replacement. *Osteoarthr. Cartil.* **2019**, *27*, 1408–1419. [CrossRef] [PubMed]
28. Hastings, D.E.; Parker, S.M. Protrusio acetabuli in rheumatoid arthritis. *Clin. Orthop. Relat. Res.* **1975**, *108*, 76–83. [CrossRef]
29. Bayley, J.C.; Christie, M.J.; Ewald, F.C.; Kelley, K. Long-term results of total hip arthroplasty in protrusio acetabuli. *J. Arthroplast.* **1987**, *2*, 275–279. [CrossRef] [PubMed]
30. Salvati, E.A.; Bullough, P.; Wilson, P.D., Jr. Intrapelvic Protrusion of the Acetabular Component Following Total Hip Replacement. *Clin. Orthop. Relat. Res.* **1975**, *111*, 212–227. [CrossRef]
31. Figueras Coll, G.; Salazar Fernandez de Erenchu, J.; Roca Burniol, J. Results of acetabular wiremesh and autograft in protrusio acetabuli. *Hip Int.* **2008**, *18*, 23–28. [CrossRef]
32. Baghdadi, Y.M.; Larson, A.N.; Sierra, R.J. Restoration of the hip center during THA performed for protrusio acetabuli is associated with better implant survival. *Clin. Orthop. Relat. Res.* **2013**, *471*, 3251–3259. [CrossRef]
33. Ansari, S.; Gupta, K.; Gupta, T.; Raja, B.S.; Pranav, J.; Kalia, R.B. Total Hip Arthroplasty in Protrusio Acetabuli: A Systematic Review. *Hip Pelvis* **2024**, *36*, 12–25. [CrossRef]
34. Rosenberg, W.W.; Schreurs, B.W.; de Waal Malefijt, M.C.; Veth, R.P.; Slooff, T.J. Impacted morsellized bone grafting and cemented primary total hip arthroplasty for acetabular protrusion in patients with rheumatoid arthritis: An 8- to 18-year follow-up study of 36 hips. *Acta Orthop. Scand.* **2000**, *71*, 143–146. [CrossRef]
35. Mibe, J.; Imakiire, A.; Watanabe, T.; Fujie, T. Results of total hip arthroplasty with bone graft and support ring for protrusio acetabuli in rheumatoid arthritis. *J. Orthop. Sci.* **2005**, *10*, 8–14. [CrossRef]
36. Unger, A.S.; Stronach, B.M.; Bergin, P.F.; Nogler, M. Direct anterior total hip arthroplasty. *Instr. Course Lect.* **2014**, *63*, 227–238.
37. Thaler, M.; Dammerer, D.; Leitner, H.; Lindtner, R.A.; Nogler, M. Mid-term Follow-up of the Direct Anterior Approach in Acetabular Revision Hip Arthroplasty Using a Reconstruction Cage With Impaction Grafting. *J. Arthroplast.* **2020**, *35*, 1339–1343. [CrossRef]
38. Prodinger, P.M.; Lazic, I.; Horas, K.; Burgkart, R.; von Eisenhart-Rothe, R.; Weissenberger, M.; Rudert, M.; Holzapfel, B.M. Revision Arthroplasty Through the Direct Anterior Approach Using an Asymmetric Acetabular Component. *J. Clin. Med.* **2020**, *9*, 3031. [CrossRef]
39. Abdel, M.P.; Berry, D.J. Current Practice Trends in Primary Hip and Knee Arthroplasties Among Members of the American Association of Hip and Knee Surgeons: A Long-Term Update. *J. Arthroplast.* **2019**, *34*, S24–S27. [CrossRef] [PubMed]
40. Meermans, G.; Konan, S.; Das, R.; Volpin, A.; Haddad, F.S. The direct anterior approach in total hip arthroplasty. *Bone Jt. J.* **2017**, *99-B*, 732–740. [CrossRef] [PubMed]
41. Wang, Z.; Hou, J.-Z.; Wu, C.-H.; Zhou, Y.-J.; Gu, X.-M.; Wang, H.-H.; Feng, W.; Cheng, Y.-X.; Sheng, X.; Bao, H.-W. A systematic review and meta-analysis of direct anterior approach versus posterior approach in total hip arthroplasty. *J. Orthop. Surg. Res.* **2018**, *13*, 229. [CrossRef]
42. Awad, M.E.; Farley, B.J.; Mostafa, G.; Saleh, K.J. Direct anterior approach has short-term functional benefit and higher resource requirements compared with the posterior approach in primary total hip arthroplasty. *Bone Jt. J.* **2021**, *103-B*, 1078–1087. [CrossRef]

Disclaimer/Publisher's Note: The statements, opinions and data contained in all publications are solely those of the individual author(s) and contributor(s) and not of MDPI and/or the editor(s). MDPI and/or the editor(s) disclaim responsibility for any injury to people or property resulting from any ideas, methods, instructions or products referred to in the content.

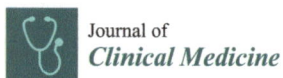

Article

Local Infiltration Analgesia Is Superior to Regional Nerve Blocks for Total Hip Arthroplasty: Less Falls, Better Mobility, and Same-Day Discharge

Catalina Baez [1,*], Hernan A. Prieto [1], Abtahi Tishad [2], Terrie Vasilopoulos [2], Emilie N. Miley [1], Justin T. Deen [3], Chancellor F. Gray [3], Hari K. Parvataneni [3] and Luis Pulido [3,*]

[1] Department of Orthopaedic Surgery and Sports Medicine, University of Florida, Gainesville, FL 32607, USA; prieth@ortho.ufl.edu (H.A.P.); emilie.miley1@gmail.com (E.N.M.)
[2] College of Medicine, University of Florida, Gainesville, FL 32607, USA; tishad100@ufl.edu (A.T.); tvasilopoulos@anest.ufl.edu (T.V.)
[3] Florida Orthopaedic Institute, Gainesville, FL 32607, USA; deenju812@gmail.com (J.T.D.); chancellor.gray@gmail.com (C.F.G.); hparvataneni@floridaortho.com (H.K.P.)
* Correspondence: baezc@ortho.ufl.edu (C.B.); luispulidos@yahoo.com (L.P.)

Abstract: Background: Multimodal analgesia in total hip arthroplasty (THA) provides better pain control, mobility, and reduced side effects compared to monotherapies. Local infiltration analgesia (LIA) and regional nerve blocks (RNBs) are commonly used throughout these protocols. This study aimed to compare these procedures as part of a multimodal analgesia protocol for patients undergoing THA. **Materials and Methods**: A retrospective review of 1100 consecutive elective primary THAs was performed in 996 patients between June 2018 and December 2021. The RNB consisted of a preoperative continuous femoral nerve catheter and single-shot obturator nerve block, and LIA consisted of the intraoperative infiltration of weight-based bupivacaine. **Results**: A total of 579 (52.6%) patients received RNB, and 521 (47.4%) received LIA. Mean oral morphine equivalents (OMEs) during the first four hours postoperatively were significantly lower for LIA group ($p < 0.001$). However, the numeric pain rating scale in the post-anesthesia care unit (PACU) was similar between groups. Patients with LIA had significantly greater first ambulation distance in the PACU ($p < 0.001$), higher successful same-day discharge rate ($p = 0.029$), fewer falls ($p = 0.041$), and less refill OMEs post-discharge ($p < 0.001$) than RNB. **Conclusions**: In the setting of similar pain management between groups and better functional outcomes for LIA, the use of minimally invasive procedures like LIA for pain control following THA is favorable.

Keywords: local infiltration analgesia; periarticular injection; peripheral nerve block; regional nerve block; total hip arthroplasty; multimodal pain management; same-day discharge; falls

1. Introduction

The shift towards elective same-day discharge (SDD) in total joint arthroplasty has proven to be safe, satisfactory, and cost-effective. Successful SDD programs highlight pain management strategies catering to early mobility, reduced side effects, and improved surgical workflow and patient experience [1–7]. Multimodal pain protocols have enhanced postoperative pain control [8,9], leveraging the synergistic effect of different analgesics to provide multifaceted pain management [10–12]. These protocols include anesthesia, preemptive analgesia, regional nerve blocks (RNBs), local infiltration analgesia (LIA), cryotherapy, and oral pain medications [8,13–15].

Regional nerve blocks consist of the preoperative infiltration of a local anesthetic around a regional nerve, achieving analgesia at the risk of motor blockade [16–19]. The placement of a catheter allows for the continuous infusion of analgesics into the perineural space which provides prolonged pain control until catheter removal upwards of three to four days later [15,20,21]. Although RNBs have consistently demonstrated to be successful at controlling postoperative pain in total hip arthroplasty (THA) [10,13,16,17], the use for proximal lower limb surgery is sub-optimal as an association has been identified with motor weakness and increased risk of falls in the postoperative period [16,18,22]. An alternative to RNB is LIA, which consists of the systematic intraoperative infiltration of a local anesthetic mixture into the periarticular tissue [14,23]. Frequently, LIA is used in THA and provides adequate pain management and patient satisfaction [15,24–26]. However, the effects of LIA are tied to the technique used and the local anesthetic cocktail of choice [23,27].

Local infiltration analgesia and periarticular injections are the most frequent methods for analgesia used in contemporary THA [18–20]. The present institution's standard of care transitioned from RNB to LIA for early postoperative pain management of THA. As such, the aim of this study was to evaluate the impact of this change on pain and functional outcomes in patients undergoing a primary THA. The primary objective was to determine whether pain outcomes (i.e., opioid requirements and pain levels in the post-anesthesia care unit [PACU] and opioids prescribed at discharge) differ between the RNB and LIA intervention. The secondary objective was to determine if functional measures (i.e., first ambulation distance, early falls, and analgesic complications) differ between groups. Finally, the tertiary objective was to compare the rate of successful SDD between groups. The hypotheses were 1.) LIA would manage postoperative pain as effectively as RNB, and 2.) LIA would allow patients to have better mobility and functional outcomes in the immediate postoperative period.

2. Materials and Methods

After Institutional Review Board approval was obtained under IRB202200276, a retrospective review was performed on patients who underwent primary THA at a single large tertiary-care academic institution. Patients were included in this study if they underwent a primary THA (i.e., CPT 27130) by one of seven fellowship-trained arthroplasty surgeons between 1 June 2018 and 31 December 2021. Patients were excluded from the study if non-arthroplasty surgeons performed their THA, had a femoral neck fracture, or received other postoperative pain management interventions.

2.1. Perioperative Planning and Medication Protocol

All cases received either 1.) intraoperative LIA by the arthroplasty surgeon or 2.) preoperative ultrasound-guided RNB with a continuous femoral nerve block catheter and portable pump for patient-controlled analgesia, paired with a single injection obturator nerve block performed preoperatively by a fellowship-trained regional and acute pain anesthesiologist. Intraoperative LIA consisted of the infiltration of weight-based bupivacaine at 0.25%. The adjusted patient body weight in kilograms was used as a reference for the volume of bupivacaine injected. A continuous femoral nerve block loading dose of 10 to 20 cc of ropivacaine 0.25% was used with a continued infusion rate at 6–8 mL per hour and patient-controlled regional analgesia boluses of 5 cc. The obturator nerve block single shots utilized 10 to 20 cc of ropivacaine at 0.25%. The surgical approach was dependent on surgeon preference and expertise. An anticipated discharge plan (i.e., same-day or inpatient) was a shared decision between the surgeon and the patient, determined by the patient's physical condition, comorbidities, and social support. The anesthesiology team determined each patient's type of intraoperative anesthesia (i.e., general or spinal).

The perioperative protocol remained consistent during this period with exception of the change from RNB to LIA. Medications used as part of multimodal pain management included preoperative dexamethasone 4–8 milligrams (mg) IV immediately before incision for postoperative nausea and single-dose postoperative ketorolac 15 mg IV; while in the PACU, medications varied and were dependent on the patient's kidney function and associated comorbidities. Postoperatively, oral medications included Tylenol 500 mg every six hours with a maximum 3000 mg per day, celecoxib 100 mg every 12 h for two weeks, and gabapentin 100 mg every night for two weeks for patients under 70 years of age with a low risk of postoperative delirium.

Additionally, oral opioid medications were prescribed according to a previously defined preoperative opioid stratification protocol; patients were categorized into one of four groups according to self-reported opioid use history: 1.) Opioid Sparing, 2.) Opioid Naïve, 3.) Standard, and 4.) Long-Term Use [28]. Opioid Sparing patients received 21 tablets of Tramadol 50 mg every 6 h as needed, Opioid Naïve patients received 28 tablets of Hydrocodone–Acetaminophen 5–325 mg every four hours as needed, Standard patients received 28 tablets of Oxycodone 5 mg every four hours as needed, and Long-Term Use patients received 21 tablets of Tramadol 50 mg every six hours as needed and 28 tablets of Oxycodone 5 mg every four hours as needed and were instructed to continue the prescribed baseline opioid treatment.

2.2. Outcomes

Relevant demographic (i.e., age, body mass index [BMI], American Society of Anesthesiologist [ASA] scores, sex, history of anxiety, history of depression, chronic preoperative opioid use, and opioid stratification pathway) and perioperative (e.g., anesthesia type, surgical approach, length of stay [LOS]) data were collected. Of note, patients were classified as "Chronic Opioid Users" when prescribed opioid medication 30 days before surgery. Similarly, classification based on the preoperative opioid stratification protocol categorized patients as "Long-Term Use" [28]. However, discrepancies were noted between these two classifications. The numeric pain rating scale (NRS) was recorded by the nursing and physical therapy staff in the PACU. The NRS is intended to assess the patient's pain on a scale from zero to ten, where zero represented no pain and ten represented the worst pain imaginable [29,30].

Opioids administered were converted into oral morphine equivalents (OMEs) according to the Centers for Disease Control Oral Morphine Milligram Equivalents conversion factors [31], which allows for standardized comparisons between groups. The primary outcome of interest was the total sum of OMEs received in the PACU and the hourly sum of OMEs during the first four hours. Secondary pain outcomes collected in the PACU included the sum of IV-only OMEs, rate of rescue opioids, total and hourly average NRS in the first four hours postoperatively, and rate of rescue nerve blocks administered for breakthrough postoperative pain. Pre- and postoperative opioid prescription and refill data were collected as OMEs. Functional outcomes were first ambulation distance (FAD), postanesthetic complications recorded in the PACU, the rate of early falls (i.e., all falls reported during the first seven days postoperatively), and successful SDD rate (i.e., the rate of patients planned for SDD that were successfully discharged on the same calendar day).

2.3. Statistical Analysis

Statistical analyses were performed using the statistical software IBM SPSS version 28. Categorical measures were summarized with counts and percentages, and continuous measures were summarized using means and standard deviations (SDs). Categorical variables were analyzed for between-group comparisons with chi-square and Fisher's exact tests. Given the large sample size, parametric tests were used for non-normally distributed single-measurement variables [32]. Single-measurement continuous variables were compared using independent t-tests or analysis of variance (ANOVA). Post hoc multivariable analyses were used to control confounders for between-group (i.e., RNB, LIA) differences for the outcomes with significant results.

Repeated measures were analyzed using generalized linear mixed modeling (GLMM) for a negative binomial distribution with pairwise comparisons and adjusted for multiple comparisons with Sidak correction. Generalized linear mixed modeling is a type of statistical analysis that allows for the development of fixed and random effect regression models that use multilevel continuous and categorical variables regardless of distributions and repeated measures, correcting for non-normality and covariance in the data [32]. Given the non-normal distribution of the repeated measures analyzed and the increased missing data after hour four in the PACU, GLMM was the most appropriate statistical test. In these models, we individually evaluated the fixed effects of time and intervention (RNB vs. LIA) and their interaction on hourly OMEs and the NRS in the PACU. Statistical significance was set to $p < 0.05$.

3. Results

A total of 1455 THA cases were identified between 1 June 2018 and 31 December 2021. However, 355 cases were excluded from the study due to the following reasons: 1.) 15 patients had a THA performed by a non-arthroplasty-specific surgeon, 2.) 105 patients had a femoral neck fracture, and 3.) 235 patients received other pain management interventions. The final sample included 1100 THA cases across 996 patients. Of these, 579 cases (52.6%) received RNB and 521 cases (47.4%) received LIA. Demographic characteristics in the population were generally balanced, except for differences between RNB and LIA for sex ($p = 0.042$), ASA scores ($p < 0.001$), depression ($p = 0.031$), and anticipated discharge plan ($p < 0.001$, Table 1).

Table 1. Patient demographics.

	Total N = 1100	RNB n = 579	LIA n = 521	*p*-Value *
Age, mean (SD)	65 (11.1)	64 (11)	65 (11)	0.185
BMI, mean (SD)	31 (7.5)	31 (7)	31 (8)	0.413
Sex, n (%)				0.042
Male	482 (43.8)	237 (40.9)	245 (47.0)	
Female	618 (56.2)	342 (59.1)	276 (53.0)	
ASA Score, n (%)				<0.001
1	4 (0.4)	2 (0.3)	2 (0.4)	
2	360 (32.7)	157 (27.1)	203 (39.0)	
3	712 (64.8)	412 (71.2)	300 (57.6)	
4	24 (2.2)	8 (1.4)	16 (3.1)	
Anxiety Diagnosis, n (%)	405 (36.8)	215 (37.1)	190 (36.5)	0.819
Depression Diagnosis, n (%)	328 (29.8)	189 (32.6)	139 (26.7)	**0.031**
Preoperative Opioid Stratification, n (%)				0.542
Opioid Sparing	52 (4.7)	31 (5.4)	21 (4.0)	
Narcotic Naïve	803 (73.0)	411 (71.0)	392 (75.2)	
Standard	120 (10.9)	68 (11.7)	52 (10.0)	
Long-Term Use	100 (9.1)	54 (9.3)	46 (8.8)	
Chronic Opioid User, n (%)	181 (16.5)	86 (14.9)	95 (18.2)	0.131
Anticipated Discharge Plan, n (%)				**<0.001**
Inpatient	745 (68.0)	508 (88.3)	237 (45.5)	
Same-day discharge	351 (32.0)	67 (11.7)	284 (54.5)	

Abbreviations: RNB: regional nerve block, LIA: local infiltration analgesia, BMI: body mass index, ASA Score: American Society of Anesthesiologists Physical Status Classification. * All bolded *p*-values indicate a statistically significant difference at $p < 0.05$.

Several perioperative factors (Table 2) were identified to be significantly different between groups. First, the surgical approach was significantly different ($p < 0.001$), with a larger proportion of posterior approach in the RNB. Similarly, RNB inpatients had significantly more extended stays in the PACU than LIA inpatients ($p < 0.001$). However, differences in type of anesthesia, surgical time, LOS, and duration in the PACU for SDD patients were not significantly different between groups.

Table 2. Perioperative outcomes.

	Total N = 1100	RNB n = 579	LIA n = 521	p-Value *
Type of Intraoperative Anesthesia, n (%)				0.096
General	854 (77.6)	461 (79.6)	393 (75.4)	
Spinal	246 (22.4)	118 (20.4)	128 (24.6)	
Surgical Approach, n (%)				**<0.001**
Anterolateral	14 (1.3)	13 (2.2)	1 (0.0)	
Direct anterior	319 (29.0)	139 (24.0)	180 (34.5)	
Posterior	767 (69.7)	427 (73.7)	340 (65.3)	
Duration of surgery (mins), mean (SD)				
Same-day discharge	87.0 (20.0)	89 (20.0)	86 (20.0)	0.832
Inpatient	98.4 (29.4)	95 (28.0)	98 (29.0)	0.192
Time in PACU (hours), mean (SD)				
Same-day discharge	5.0 (1.4)	5.2 (1.4)	4.9 (1.4)	0.930
Inpatient	4.5 (3.4)	4.6 (3.0)	4.5 (3.3)	**<0.001**
Length of stay (hours), mean (SD)				
Same-day discharge	9.3 (1.9)	9.5 (2.2)	9.28 (1.8)	1.000
Inpatient	55.9 (37.2)	43.9 (38.0)	52.24 (37.8)	0.625

Abbreviations: RNB: regional nerve block, LIA: local infiltration analgesia, PACU: post-anesthesia care unit. * All bolded p-values indicate a statistically significant difference at p < 0.05.

As differences were identified among groups at baseline (i.e., sex, ASA score, depression, and anticipated discharge plan), we performed multivariable analyses to control for baseline differences. No confounding effects were identified between the covariates and the main effect of the interventions (i.e., RNB and LIA) with p-values ranging from 0.125 to 0.971.

3.1. Pain Outcomes

3.1.1. Opioid Requirements

Mean OME requirements during the first four hours in the PACU were significantly different between groups ($F[1, 2220] = 11.51$, $p < 0.001$; Figure 1), where the LIA group averaged less OMEs (3.8 ± 6.6) than the RNB group (4.5 ± 7.3; $p < 0.001$). Additionally, OME requirements significantly decreased over time regardless of the group ($F[3, 2220] = 74.44$, $p < 0.001$). Although the LIA group required significantly fewer OMEs (9.5 ± 8.5) than RNB group (10.2 ± 9.1; $p = 0.002$) at hours one and three (LIA = 1.2 ± 3.7, RNB = 1.5 ± 4.1; $p = 0.020$; Figure 1), the combined effect of the groups across time on OMEs in the PACU was not statistically significant ($F[3, 2220] = 0.83$, $p = 0.478$).

The sum of intravenous opioids required in the PACU was not significantly different ($t[1093.52] = 1.47$, $p = 0.143$). However, patients in the LIA group required almost double as many OMEs as the patients in the RNB group (Table 3). In addition, there were significantly more patients in the LIA group (81.2%) that required rescue opioids in the PACU compared to the RNB group (74.1%; $\chi^2 = 7.91$, $p = 0.006$, Table 3). Patients in the LIA group had 1.5 higher odds (95% CI [1.1, 2.0]) of needing rescue opioids during their initial PACU stay than RNB patients. However, the mean sum of all OMEs received during their PACU stay was not significantly different ($t[1094.67] = 0.24$, $p = 0.809$) between the LIA (12.8 ± 10.8) and RNB (12.6 ± 12.6) groups.

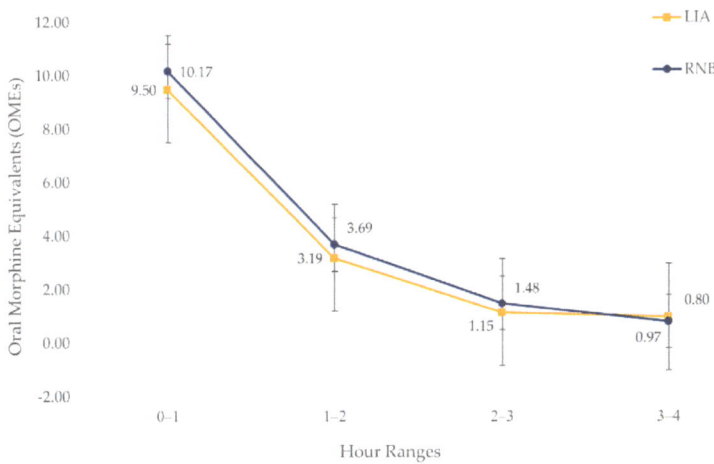

Figure 1. Mean OMEs received in PACU.

Table 3. Pain and functional outcomes.

	Total N = 1100	RNB N = 579	LIA N = 521	*p*-Value *
Pain Outcomes				
Rate of opioids received in PACU, (%)	852 (77.5)	429 (74.1)	423 (81.2)	**0.005**
Total OMEs in PACU, mean (SD)	12.7 (11.8)	12.6 (12.6)	12.8 (10.7)	0.809
Rescue IV OMEs in PACU, mean (SD)	9.2 (51.0)	6.9 (14.2)	11.7 (72.5)	0.143
Rate of rescue nerve blocks in PACU, n (%)	20 (1.8)	14 (2.4)	6 (1.2)	0.117
Prescribed OMEs, mean (SD)				0.938
Total	395.9 (642.7)	396.2 (574.0)	396.2 (711.9)	
Daily	4.4 (7.1)	4.4 (6.0)	4.4 (7.9)	
Postoperative opioid refills (90 d), mean (SD)				
Number of refills	1.4 (0.8)	1.4 (0.7)	1.4 (0.9)	0.716
Total refill OMEs	221.1 (160.9)	282.2 (182.1)	176.7 (126.9)	**<0.001**
Daily refill OMEs	2.5 (1.7)	3.1 (2.0)	1.96 (1.4)	**<0.001**
Functional outcomes				
Postanesthetic complications, n (%)	73 (6.6)	38 (6.6)	35 (6.7)	0.918
FAD in PACU (ft), mean (SD)	31.2 (55.1)	22 (37.0)	42 (68.0)	**<0.001**
Successful same-day discharge rate, n (%)	310/351 (88.3)	54/67 (80.6)	256/284 (90.1)	**0.029**
Early falls, n (%)	12 (1.1)	10 (1.7)	2 (0.4)	**0.041**

Abbreviations: RNB: regional nerve block, LIA: local infiltration analgesia, PACU: post-anesthesia care unit, OMEs: oral morphine equivalents, IV: intravenous, FAD: first ambulation distance. * All bolded *p*-values indicate a statistically significant difference.

The rate of rescue nerve blocks required in the PACU (n = 20) was twice as high in the RNB group (2.4%, n = 14) than in the LIA group (1.2%, n = 6, Table 3), though this difference was not statistically significant ($\chi^2 = 2.46$, $p = 0.174$). The most frequently performed rescue nerve block was a single-shot lateral femoral cutaneous nerve block (35%, n = 7), followed by combination blocks with more than one targeted nerve (30%, n = 6). The remaining 35% (n = 7) of the rescue blocks performed were one single-shot pectineus nerve block, one single-shot sciatic nerve block, two pericapsular nerve group blocks, two field blocks, and one epidural block.

Lastly, the mean OME refills were significantly different between groups (t[195] = −4.5, $p < 0.001$), with patients in the RNB group receiving more opioids (282.2 ± 182.1) than LIA group (176.7 ± 126.9). However, OMEs prescribed preoperatively for post-discharge pain were not significantly different between groups (t[998.80] = 0.002, p = 0.999), with patients in the LIA group having a mean of 396.2 ± 711.9 OMEs for the first 90 days (i.e., average of 4.4 ± 7.9 per day) and the RNB group having a mean of 396.2 ± 574.0 OMEs for the first 90 days (i.e., average of 4.4 ± 6.4 per day).

3.1.2. Numeric Pain Rating Scale

The average NRS recorded for patients in the PACU did not significantly differ between groups (t[1093.52] = 1.66, p = 0.097), with patients in the LIA group having a mean score of 4.2 ± 2.4 compared to a mean score of 4.0 ±2.6 in the RNB group. Additionally, the mean NRS recorded during the first four hours in the PACU was not significantly different for either group (F[1, 3459] = 3.07, p = 0.080). Pain levels reported in the PACU significantly decreased over time (F[3, 3459] = 23.37, p < 0.001). The combined effect of the group and time on the mean hourly NRS in the PACU showed an overall significant difference (F[3, 3459] = 3.08, p = 0.027), specifically at hour two (LIA = 4.4 ± 2.7, RNB = 4.0 ± 3.0; p = 0.014) and hour three (LIA = 4.0 ± 2.5, RNB = 3.5 ± 2.8; p = 0.014; Figure 2).

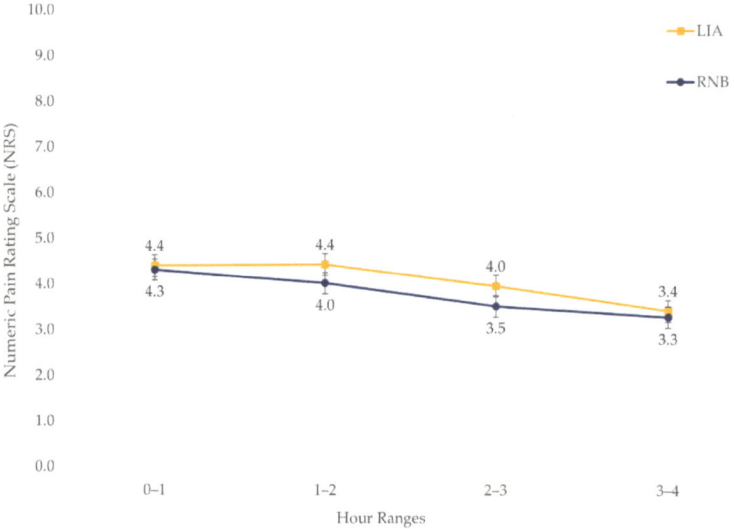

Figure 2. Mean hourly NRS recorded in PACU.

3.2. Functional Outcomes

The first ambulation distance in the PACU was significantly greater (t[611.85] = 5.10, p < 0.001) for patients in the LIA group (41.7 ft ± 68.5 ft) than RNB group (22.2 ft ± 38.3 ft). Notably, 40 patients in the RNB group could not ambulate in the PACU due to quadriceps weakness, while only three patients in the LIA group encountered a similar situation. Patients who received an RNB reported significantly (p = 0.041) more falls (1.7%, n = 10) compared to those who received LIA (0.4%, n = 2). This translated to 4.6 higher odds (95% CIs: 1.0–20.9) of falling during the first seven days after THA for patients managed with RNB over those with LIA. Postanesthetic complications recorded in the PACU were not significantly different between groups (χ^2 = 0.01, p = 0.918), with 6.6% reported for the LIA group, and 6.7% reported for the RNB group. Finally, the rate of successful SDD was significantly greater (χ^2 = 4.79, p = 0.029) in LIA (90.1%) than in RNB (80.6%). Thus, of those patients who were anticipated to have an SDD, those who received LIA had 2.2 higher odds (95% CIs: 1.07–4.5) of being successfully discharged on the same day than patients who received RNB.

4. Discussion

Increasing demand for adequate postoperative pain management that avoids motor blockade and allows for early patient mobilization has led to the quick adoption of LIA for immediate postoperative pain management in patients undergoing THA. Although multiple studies have compared the efficacy of LIA and different regional nerve blocks on postoperative pain after THA [14,15,22,24–26,33,34], only few studies have compared the effects of these interventions during the immediate postoperative period [14,25,26]. Additionally, modern SDD Enhanced Recovery After Surgery (ERAS) protocols must factor in baseline patient function, safety, and pain control, as most patients are now out of the hospital setting during early recovery. Consequently, our study aimed to determine if there was a difference in pain and functional outcomes between LIA and RNB for THA during the patient's stay in the PACU.

Patients consumed less OMEs across time spent in the PACU which suggests that opioid requirements decreased significantly during the first four hours after surgery regardless of the intervention groups. Fewer patients in the RNB group required opioids in the PACU than patients in the LIA group, which demonstrates 1.5 higher odds of requiring rescue opioids during this time. However, the sum of OMEs received remained the same between groups. Patients in the RNB group received double the rate of rescue nerve blocks than LIA patients, although this difference was not statistically significant. Furthermore, RNB patients had access to patient-controlled analgesia via the continuous femoral nerve block, introducing a pain-controlling pathway that LIA patients lacked. As such, the clinical effect of LIA and RNB on opioid requirements in the immediate postoperative period was similar, underscoring the consideration of each patient's functional goals in deciding between these two interventions [24].

Preoperatively prescribed OMEs for postoperative pain did not differ between groups, reflecting the arthroplasty division's efforts to standardize opioid prescription in compliance with state and federal laws [28]. Demographic data obtained demonstrated a balance across opioid stratification of patients, and unsurprisingly, records of prescribed OMEs were similar between groups. The OME conversions for opioid refills given during the first 90 days after surgery work as a surrogate for pain management beyond hospitalization. Continuous RNB patients consumed greater amounts of opioids during this period, contradicting the theoretical concept of prolonged analgesia for RNB [20–22].

The average NRS in the PACU was similar between groups, but decreased significantly across time achieving a minimal clinically important difference of one point between hours one and four [29,30]. Whether this is due to the interventions under analysis, the consumed opioids in the PACU, or the natural history of pain in the postoperative period is unclear from this dataset. However, findings from this study are comparable to other authors who have identified similar pain control between LIA and RNB groups [25,35–37]. Postanesthetic complications did not differ between groups which may reflect the balance in types of anesthesia used and opioids consumed across groups, which other authors have also identified similar findings [14,15,22,25,26,37]. Given that RNB and LIA provide similar levels of pain control, functional outcomes may have a greater weight in directing pain management. First, ambulation distance reflects adequate pain control and directly influences early discharge in total joint arthroplasty [3]. Within this study sample, LIA patients ambulated an average of 20 ft more than RNB patients in the PACU, with more RNB patients reporting quadricep weakness as the cause of ambulation failure. Similarly, falls soon after surgery are an essential indicator of functional capacity after THA. Patients in this study who received an RNB had 4.6 higher odds of having a fall within the first week after surgery than those who received LIA. Two of the RNB patients who fell associated the event with quadriceps weakness. On the contrary, LIA patients only reported two falls due to slip and fall. These findings are supported by a previous systematic review and meta-analysis which identified continuous lumbar plexus block associated with an increased risk of falls compared to single-shot lumbar plexus block, wherein this type of block also targets the femoral and obturator nerves used by our team [18]. Furthermore, the

American Association of Hip and Knee Surgeons, the American Academy of Orthopedic Surgery, the American Society of Regional Anesthesia and Pain Management, the Hip Society, and the Knee Society combined safety and efficacy panel has recently advised against continuous and single-shot femoral nerve blocks due to their increased risk of motor weakness [22].

Finally, the successful SDD rate was significantly greater in patients who obtained a LIA than RNB, where the LIA group had 2.2 higher odds of achieving SDD. For SDD to be completed, patients had to ambulate safely, have well-controlled pain, no vomiting or nausea, and have normal bladder function. Since pain levels and complication rates are not different between interventions, the primary catalyst for successful SDD may be related to factors that allow for improved ambulation in the PACU. A previous study in the present institution found that longer first ambulation distances were associated with successful SDD [3], further supporting pain management techniques that spare muscle function, such as LIA.

This study is not without its limitations. First, as this study was retrospective in nature, inherent difficulties existed in data collection and analysis. However, the statistical analyses used attempted to consider these structural limitations and control for them. Second, there were baseline differences between groups in terms of sex, ASA score, depression rates, anticipated discharge plan, and surgical approach. However, post-hoc multivariable regression was performed to control for these differences and assess the confounding effect on the significant outcomes. No variables were identified to significantly confound the expected impact of the intervention on the outcomes. However, this study may have been underpowered to address these confounding effects, and the results should be interpreted considering these differences; as female sex, depression diagnoses, and surgical approach have been conflictingly associated with higher levels of postoperative pain [38–43]. Regardless, these data demonstrated similar pain levels and opioid requirements between groups.

Third, although not statistically significant, there is a general trend toward increased use of spinal anesthesia over general anesthesia, potentially introducing bias to the data. The dose of spinal anesthesia and the adjuvants used has been reported to significantly affect pain management, LOS, and complications after hip surgery which could confound the effects of RNB and LIA on pain and functional outcomes [8,44–47]. Nonetheless, the protocols for ERAS favor using spinal anesthesia for SDD management [48]. Ultimately, these differences noted between groups reflect changes adopted over time by the anesthesia and arthroplasty departments for preferred patient management practices. Fourth, the transition to LIA was shortly followed by the 2020 coronavirus pandemic and Medicare's exclusion of THA from the inpatient-only list. This led to an increased volume of SDD THAs, echoed by the significant differences amongst groups for anticipated discharge plans. However, these changes did not affect the pain intervention received by our patients nor the calculation for successful SDD. Fifth, although the use of a stratification pathway for opioid prescription is an excellent way to curve physician opioid over-prescribing, the existence of this pathway limits the analyzability of our data for preoperatively prescribed OMEs. It is unlikely that these were related to the pain intervention given that the prescription pathway accounts for expected opioid needs at home regardless of the planned perioperative pain management strategy [28]. Data on refills better represent the effect of OMEs required postoperatively. Lastly, this was a single-institution series, potentially limiting the generalizability of the data. This was partially compensated for by the inclusion of THAs performed by seven different fellowship-trained orthopedic surgeons, increasing the generalizability of the results. Nonetheless, this study provides the largest sample for comparison to date.

5. Conclusions

Data comparing LIA and RNB interventions as immediate postoperative pain management methods demonstrated minimal differences in objective and subjective pain measures. Additionally, this study provided further evidence that postoperative pain after THA is adequately controlled with less invasive procedures such as LIA. Functional outcomes analyzed in this study support using LIA over RNB as patients who received this treatment had increased first ambulation distance, greater odds of a successful SDD, fewer postoperative falls, and similar pain outcomes to RNB. As such, these findings further support using LIA for primary elective THA.

Author Contributions: Conceptualization, L.P., C.B., H.A.P., J.T.D., C.F.G. and H.K.P.; methodology, C.B. and L.P.; validation, C.B. and T.V.; formal analysis, C.B. and T.V.; investigation, C.B. and L.P.; data curation, C.B.; writing—original draft preparation, C.B., A.T. and L.P.; writing—review and editing, H.A.P., E.N.M., J.T.D., C.F.G. and H.K.P.; visualization, C.B.; supervision, L.P.; project administration, E.N.M. All authors have read and agreed to the published version of the manuscript.

Funding: This research received no external funding.

Institutional Review Board Statement: The study was conducted per the Declaration of Helsinki and approved by the Institutional Review Board of the University of Florida (protocol IRB202200276 on 17 February 2022).

Informed Consent Statement: Patient consent was waived because this study was a retrospective chart review.

Data Availability Statement: The dataset analyzed during the study is not publicly available per the study protocol. De-identified data may be available from the corresponding author with permission from the University of Florida upon reasonable request.

Conflicts of Interest: The authors declare no conflicts of interest.

References

1. Bertin, K.C. Minimally invasive outpatient total hip arthroplasty: A financial analysis. *Clin. Orthop. Relat. Res.* **2005**, *435*, 154–163. [CrossRef] [PubMed]
2. Dorr, L.D.; Thomas, D.J.; Zhu, J.; Dastane, M.; Chao, L.; Long, W.T. Outpatient total hip arthroplasty. *J. Arthroplast.* **2010**, *25*, 501–506. [CrossRef] [PubMed]
3. Gogineni, H.C.; Gray, C.F.; Prieto, H.A.; Deen, J.T.; Boezaart, A.P.; Parvataneni, H.K. Transition to outpatient total hip and knee arthroplasty: Experience at an academic tertiary care center. *Arthroplast. Today* **2019**, *5*, 100–105. [CrossRef] [PubMed]
4. Goyal, N.; Chen, A.F.; Padgett, S.E.; Tan, T.L.; Kheir, M.M.; Hopper, R.H.; Hamilton, W.G.; Hozack, W.J. Otto Aufranc Award: A Multicenter, Randomized Study of Outpatient versus Inpatient Total Hip Arthroplasty. *Clin. Orthop. Relat. Res.* **2017**, *475*, 364–372. [CrossRef] [PubMed]
5. Hoffmann, J.D.; Kusnezov, N.A.; Dunn, J.C.; Zarkadis, N.J.; Goodman, G.P.; Berger, R.A. The Shift to Same-Day Outpatient Joint Arthroplasty: A Systematic Review. *J. Arthroplast.* **2018**, *33*, 1265–1274. [CrossRef] [PubMed]
6. Kelly, M.P.; Calkins, T.E.; Culvern, C.; Kogan, M.; Della Valle, C.J. Inpatient versus outpatient hip and knee arthroplasty: Which has higher patient satisfaction? *J. Arthroplast.* **2018**, *33*, 3402–3406. [CrossRef] [PubMed]
7. Rosinsky, P.J.; Go, C.C.; Bheem, R.; Shapira, J.; Maldonado, D.R.; Meghpara, M.B.; Lall, A.C.; Domb, B.G. The cost-effectiveness of outpatient surgery for primary total hip arthroplasty in the United States: A computer-based cost-utility study. *Hip Int.* **2021**, *31*, 572–581. [CrossRef] [PubMed]
8. Parvizi, J.; Miller, A.G.; Gandhi, K. Multimodal pain management after total joint arthroplasty. *J. Bone Jt. Surg. Am.* **2011**, *93*, 1075–1084. [CrossRef]
9. Helander, E.M.; Menard, B.L.; Harmon, C.M.; Homra, B.K.; Allain, A.V.; Bordelon, G.J.; Wyche, M.Q.; Padnos, I.W.; Lavrova, A.; Kaye, A.D. Multimodal analgesia, current concepts, and acute pain considerations. *Curr. Pain Headache Rep.* **2017**, *21*, 3. [CrossRef]
10. Grant, C.R.K.; Checketts, M.R. Analgesia for primary hip and knee arthroplasty: The role of regional anaesthesia. *Contin. Educ. Anaesth. Crit. Care Pain* **2008**, *8*, 56–61. [CrossRef]
11. Ranawat, A.S.; Ranawat, C.S. Pain management and accelerated rehabilitation for total hip and total knee arthroplasty. *J. Arthroplast.* **2007**, *22* (Suppl. 3), 12–15. [CrossRef] [PubMed]
12. Chou, R.; Gordon, D.B.; de Leon-Casasola, O.A.; Rosenberg, J.M.; Bickler, S.; Brennan, T.; Carter, T.; Cassidy, C.L.; Chittenden, E.H.; Degenhardt, E.; et al. Management of postoperative pain: A clinical practice guideline from the american pain society, the american society of regional anesthesia and pain medicine, and the american society of anesthesiologists' committee on regional anesthesia, executive committee, and administrative council. *J. Pain* **2016**, *17*, 131–157. [CrossRef]
13. Pagnano, M.W.; Hebl, J.; Horlocker, T. Assuring a painless total hip arthroplasty: A multimodal approach emphasizing peripheral nerve blocks. *J. Arthroplast.* **2006**, *21* (Suppl. 1), 80–84. [CrossRef] [PubMed]
14. Kerr, D.R.; Kohan, L. Local infiltration analgesia: A technique for the control of acute postoperative pain following knee and hip surgery: A case study of 325 patients. *Acta Orthop.* **2008**, *79*, 174–183. [CrossRef]

15. Johnson, R.L.; Amundson, A.W.; Abdel, M.P.; Sviggum, H.P.; Mabry, T.M.; Mantilla, C.B.; Schroeder, D.R.; Pagnano, M.W.; Kopp, S.L. Continuous Posterior Lumbar Plexus Nerve Block Versus Periarticular Injection with Ropivacaine or Liposomal Bupivacaine for Total Hip Arthroplasty: A Three-Arm Randomized Clinical Trial. *J. Bone Jt. Surg. Am.* **2017**, *99*, 1836–1845. [CrossRef]
16. Stein, B.E.; Srikumaran, U.; Tan, E.W.; Freehill, M.T.; Wilckens, J.H. Lower-extremity peripheral nerve blocks in the perioperative pain management of orthopaedic patients: AAOS exhibit selection. *J. Bone Jt. Surg. Am.* **2012**, *94*, e167. [CrossRef]
17. Guay, J.; Johnson, R.L.; Kopp, S. Nerve blocks or no nerve blocks for pain control after elective hip replacement (arthroplasty) surgery in adults. *Cochrane Database Syst. Rev.* **2017**, *10*, CD011608. [CrossRef] [PubMed]
18. Johnson, R.L.; Kopp, S.L.; Hebl, J.R.; Erwin, P.J.; Mantilla, C.B. Falls and major orthopaedic surgery with peripheral nerve blockade: A systematic review and meta-analysis. *Br. J. Anaesth.* **2013**, *110*, 518–528. [CrossRef]
19. Horlocker, T.T.; Kopp, S.L.; Pagnano, M.W.; Hebl, J.R. Analgesia for total hip and knee arthroplasty: A multimodal pathway featuring peripheral nerve block. *J. Am. Acad. Orthop. Surg.* **2006**, *14*, 126–135. [CrossRef]
20. Watson, M.W.; Mitra, D.; McLintock, T.C.; Grant, S.A. Continuous versus single-injection lumbar plexus blocks: Comparison of the effects on morphine use and early recovery after total knee arthroplasty. *Reg. Anesth. Pain Med.* **2005**, *30*, 541–547. [CrossRef]
21. Ilfeld, B.M.; Gearen, P.F.; Enneking, F.K.; Berry, L.F.; Spadoni, E.H.; George, S.Z.; Vandenborne, K. Total knee arthroplasty as an overnight-stay procedure using continuous femoral nerve blocks at home: A prospective feasibility study. *Anesth. Analg.* **2006**, *102*, 87–90. [CrossRef]
22. Fillingham, Y.A.; Hannon, C.P.; Kopp, S.L.; Austin, M.S.; Sershon, R.A.; Stronach, B.M.; Meneghini, R.M.; Abdel, M.P.; Griesemer, M.E.; Woznica, A.; et al. The Efficacy and Safety of Regional Nerve Blocks in Total Knee Arthroplasty: Systematic Review and Direct Meta-Analysis. *J. Arthroplast.* **2022**, *37*, 1906–1921.e2. [CrossRef]
23. Amundson, A.W.; Panchamia, J.K.; Jacob, A.K. Anesthesia for Same-Day Total Joint Replacement. *Anesthesiol. Clin.* **2019**, *37*, 251–264. [CrossRef]
24. Jiménez-Almonte, J.H.; Wyles, C.C.; Wyles, S.P.; Norambuena-Morales, G.A.; Báez, P.J.; Murad, M.H.; Sierra, R.J. Is Local Infiltration Analgesia Superior to Peripheral Nerve Blockade for Pain Management After THA: A Network Meta-analysis. *Clin. Orthop. Relat. Res.* **2016**, *474*, 495–516. [CrossRef] [PubMed]
25. Busch, C.A.; Whitehouse, M.R.; Shore, B.J.; MacDonald, S.J.; McCalden, R.W.; Bourne, R.B. The efficacy of periarticular multimodal drug infiltration in total hip arthroplasty. *Clin. Orthop. Relat. Res.* **2010**, *468*, 2152–2159. [CrossRef]
26. Kuchálik, J.; Magnuson, A.; Lundin, A.; Gupta, A. Local infiltration analgesia or femoral nerve block for postoperative pain management in patients undergoing total hip arthroplasty. A randomized, double-blind study. *Scand. J. Pain* **2017**, *16*, 223–230. [CrossRef] [PubMed]
27. McCarthy, D.; Iohom, G. Local Infiltration Analgesia for Postoperative Pain Control following Total Hip Arthroplasty: A Systematic Review. *Anesthesiol. Res. Pract.* **2012**, *2012*, 709531. [CrossRef] [PubMed]
28. Deen, J.T.; Stone, W.Z.; Gray, C.F.; Prieto, H.A.; Iams, D.A.; Boezaart, A.P.; Parvataneni, H.K. A simple, personalized opioid stratification pathway dramatically reduces opioid utilization. *Arthroplast. Today* **2020**, *6*, 731–735. [CrossRef]
29. Salaffi, F.; Stancati, A.; Silvestri, C.A.; Ciapetti, A.; Grassi, W. Minimal clinically important changes in chronic musculoskeletal pain intensity measured on a numerical rating scale. *Eur. J. Pain* **2004**, *8*, 283–291. [CrossRef]
30. Fan, X.Y.; Ma, J.H.; Wu, X.; Xu, X.; Shi, L.; Li, T.; Wang, P.; Li, C.; Li, Z.; Zhang, Q.Y.; et al. How much improvement can satisfy patients? Exploring patients' satisfaction 3 years after total knee arthroplasty. *J. Orthop. Surg. Res.* **2021**, *16*, 389. [CrossRef]
31. US Department of Health and Human Services—Centers for Disease Control and Prevention. Calculating Total Daily Dose of Opiods for Safer Dosage. Available online: https://archive.cdc.gov/www_cdc_gov/opioids/data-resources/index.html (accessed on 13 April 2022).
32. Kwak, S.G.; Kim, J.H. Central limit theorem: The cornerstone of modern statistics. *Korean J. Anesthesiol.* **2017**, *70*, 144–156. [CrossRef] [PubMed]
33. Parvataneni, H.K.; Ranawat, A.S.; Ranawat, C.S. The use of local periarticular injections in the management of postoperative pain after total hip and knee replacement: A multimodal approach. *Instr. Course Lect.* **2007**, *56*, 125–131. [PubMed]
34. Parvataneni, H.K.; Shah, V.P.; Howard, H.; Cole, N.; Ranawat, A.S.; Ranawat, C.S. Controlling pain after total hip and knee arthroplasty using a multimodal protocol with local periarticular injections: A prospective randomized study. *J. Arthroplast.* **2007**, *22* (Suppl. 2), 33–38. [CrossRef] [PubMed]
35. Ewing, M.; Huff, H.; Heil, S.; Borsheski, R.R.; Smith, M.J.; Kim, H.M. Local infiltration analgesia versus interscalene block for pain management following shoulder arthroplasty: A prospective randomized clinical trial. *J. Bone Jt. Surg. Am.* **2022**, *104*, 1730–1737. [CrossRef]
36. Kethy, J.E.; Carrie, F.; Daniel, M.; Jacques, Y.; David, M.; Peter, S. Minimizing Opioid Use after Total Hip Arthroplasty: Comparing Periarticular Injection versus Patient Controlled Epidural Analgesia versus a Combination Protocol. *J. Arthroplast.* **2022**, *38*, 101–107. [CrossRef]
37. Peters, C.L.; Shirley, B.; Erickson, J. The effect of a new multimodal perioperative anesthetic regimen on postoperative pain, side effects, rehabilitation, and length of hospital stay after total joint arthroplasty. *J. Arthroplast.* **2006**, *21* (Suppl. 2), 132–138. [CrossRef] [PubMed]
38. Pinto, P.R.; McIntyre, T.; Ferrero, R.; Almeida, A.; Araújo-Soares, V. Predictors of acute postsurgical pain and anxiety following primary total hip and knee arthroplasty. *J. Pain* **2013**, *14*, 502–515. [CrossRef]

39. Pinto, P.R.; McIntyre, T.; Ferrero, R.; Almeida, A.; Araújo-Soares, V. Risk factors for moderate and severe persistent pain in patients undergoing total knee and hip arthroplasty: A prospective predictive study. *PLoS ONE* **2013**, *8*, e73917. [CrossRef]
40. Ip, H.Y.V.; Abrishami, A.; Peng, P.W.H.; Wong, J.; Chung, F. Predictors of postoperative pain and analgesic consumption: A qualitative systematic review. *Anesthesiology* **2009**, *111*, 657–677. [CrossRef]
41. Yang, Z.; Feng, S.; Guo, K.-J.; Zha, G.-C. Patient-reported results of simultaneous direct anterior approach and posterolateral approach total hip arthroplasties performed in the same patients. *J. Orthop. Traumatol.* **2021**, *22*, 46. [CrossRef] [PubMed]
42. Kunze, K.N.; McLawhorn, A.S.; Jules-Elysee, K.M.; Alexiades, M.M.; Desai, N.A.; Lin, Y.; Beathe, J.C.; Ma, Y.; Zhang, W.; Sculco, T.P. Effect of anterior approach compared to posterolateral approach on readiness for discharge and thrombogenic markers in patients undergoing unilateral total hip arthroplasty: A prospective cohort study. *Arch. Orthop. Trauma. Surg.* **2023**, *143*, 2217–2226. [CrossRef] [PubMed]
43. Rodriguez, S.; Shen, T.S.; Lebrun, D.G.; Della Valle, A.G.; Ast, M.P.; Rodriguez, J.A. Ambulatory total hip arthroplasty: Causes for failure to launch and associated risk factors. *Bone Jt. Open* **2022**, *3*, 684–691. [CrossRef] [PubMed]
44. Bourget-Murray, J.; Halpenny, D.; Mahdavi, S.; Piroozfar, S.G.; Sharma, R. Perioperative outcomes associated with general and spinal anesthesia after total joint arthroplasty for osteoarthritis: A large, Canadian, retrospective cohort study. *Can. J. Surg.* **2022**, *65*, E460–E467. [CrossRef] [PubMed]
45. Messina, A.; La Via, L.; Milani, A.; Savi, M.; Calabrò, L.; Sanfilippo, F.; Negri, K.; Castellani, G.; Cammarota, G.; Robba, C.; et al. Spinal anesthesia and hypotensive events in hip fracture surgical repair in elderly patients: A meta-analysis. *J. Anesth. Analg. Crit. Care* **2022**, *2*, 19. [CrossRef]
46. Wolla, C.D.; Epperson, T.I.; Woltz, E.M.; Wolf, B.J.; Bolin, E.D. Prolongation of spinal duration by escalating doses of intrathecal epinephrine in lower limb arthroplasty. *Pain Manag.* **2023**, *13*, 647–654. [CrossRef] [PubMed]
47. Yazdi, B.; Modir, H.; Kamali, A.; Masouri, H. Change in saturation oxygen and hemodynamic responses by adding intrathecal dexmedetomidine vs. sufentanil to bupivacaine in patients undergoing dynamic hip screw operation: A randomized clinical trial. *Med. Gas. Res.* **2020**, *10*, 144–148. [CrossRef]
48. Oseka, L.; Pecka, S. Anesthetic management in early recovery after surgery protocols for total knee and total hip arthroplasty. *AANA J.* **2018**, *86*, 32–39. [PubMed]

Disclaimer/Publisher's Note: The statements, opinions and data contained in all publications are solely those of the individual author(s) and contributor(s) and not of MDPI and/or the editor(s). MDPI and/or the editor(s) disclaim responsibility for any injury to people or property resulting from any ideas, methods, instructions or products referred to in the content.

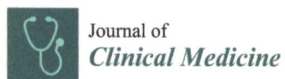

Article

Usage of Tranexamic Acid for Total Hip Arthroplasty: A Matched Cohort Analysis of 144,344 Patients

Anubhav Thapaliya [1], Mehul M. Mittal [1], Terrul L. Ratcliff [2], Varatharaj Mounasamy [2], Dane K. Wukich [2] and Senthil N. Sambandam [2,*]

[1] University of Texas Southwestern Medical School, 5323 Harry Hines Blvd, Dallas, TX 75390, USA; anubhav.thapaliya@utsouthwestern.edu (A.T.)
[2] Department of Orthopaedic Surgery, University of Texas Southwestern Medical Center, 1801 Inwood Road, Dallas, TX 75390, USA; terrul.ratcliff@utsouthwestern.edu (T.L.R.); orthovcu@gmail.com (V.M.); dane.wukich@utsouthwestern.edu (D.K.W.)
* Correspondence: sambandamortho@gmail.com; Tel.: +1-214-857-1819

Abstract: Background: The literature is inconclusive regarding the potential complications of tranexamic acid (TXA), an antifibrinolytic drug, for total hip arthroplasty (THA). The purpose of this study is to compare complication rates and patient outcomes between THA patients administered TXA vs. THA patients not administered TXA. **Methods:** The TriNetX Research network was utilized to generate a cohort of adult patients who underwent THA between 2003 and 2024. These patients were categorized into two subgroups for the retrospective analysis: (1) patients who received TXA 24 h prior to THA (TXA), and (2) patients who did not receive TXA 24 h prior to total hip arthroplasty (no-TXA). The follow-up period was 30 and 90 days. **Results:** At 30 days following THA, the TXA patients had a reduced risk of transfusion (risk ratio (RR): 0.412; 95% confidence intervals (CI): 0.374, 0.453), reduced risk of DVT (RR: 0.856; CI: 0.768, 0.953), reduced risk of joint infection (RR: 0.808; CI: 0.710, 0.920), but a higher rate of periprosthetic fracture (RR: 1.234; CI: 1.065, 1.429) compared to patients who did not receive TXA. At 90 days following THA, TXA patients had a reduced risk of transfusion (RR: 0.446; CI: 0.408, 0.487), DVT (RR: 0.847; CI: 0.776, 0.924), and periprosthetic joint infection (RR: 0.894; CI: 0.815, 0.982) compared to patients who did not receive TXA. Patients who received TXA had higher rates of periprosthetic fracture (RR: 1.219; CI: 1.088, 1.365), acute postoperative anemia (RR: 1.222; CI: 1.171, 1.276), deep surgical site infection (SSI) (RR: 1.706; CI: 1.117, 2.605), and superficial SSI (RR: 1.950; CI: 1.567, 2.428) compared to patients who did not receive TXA. **Conclusions:** Patients receiving TXA prior to THA exhibited significantly reduced the prevalence of blood transfusions, DVT, and periprosthetic joint infection following THA. However, superficial SSI and periprosthetic fracture were seen with higher rates in the TXA cohort than in the no-TXA cohort.

Keywords: tranexamic acid (TXA); total hip arthroplasty (THA); antifibrinolytics; perioperative surgery

1. Introduction

Tranexamic acid (TXA) is a synthetic drug, administered both topically and intravenously, that inhibits fibrinolysis and clot breakdown to reduce blood loss [1]. TXA can also be intravenously administered as a prophylactic measure to decrease blood loss and lower the likelihood of blood transfusion [2]. Moreover, TXA is typically administered within 24 h of a surgical procedure, as there is increased fibrinolytic activity in the first hours of surgery [3].

Total hip arthroplasty (THA) is a safe and routinely performed surgical intervention [4], with over 450,000 THA procedures performed annually in the United States (US) [5]. Primarily performed in the elderly, THA can treat the degenerative manifestations of end-stage hip joint disease as well as relieve hip joint pain and enhance the quality of life through improved joint mobility [6,7]. Projections indicate that by 2030, primary THA is expected to grow by 171%, with revision THA expected to increase by 142% in the same time frame [8]. However, despite the high prevalence of THA and 90% survivorship at 10 years [9], complications can result, ranging from periprosthetic dislocation and fractures to hematomas [10]. Postoperative complications are most common in elderly patient populations and comorbid patients [8,11], with common THA complications including blood loss and associated post-operative anemia [12]. Significant blood loss can necessitate allogenic blood transfusions, which introduces more potential complications and adverse events to the THA. Hence, research efforts are aimed at optimizing blood management to reduce transfusion rates and blood loss [13]. For example, Zhu et al. reported a statistically significant reduction in total blood loss, intraoperative blood loss, postoperative blood loss, hemoglobin drop, allogenic blood transfusion rate, and average hospital stay with TXA administration in THA when compared to controls [14].

Although the previous literature has established that TXA improves THA outcomes by reducing blood loss [15,16], the widespread adoption of TXA in the surgical community has been limited by possible side effects [3]. For example, due to its antifibrinolytic properties, TXA is regarded as an independent risk factor for venous thromboembolism [17]. Even in patients with low thrombotic risk, studies suggest a possible association between TXA administration and an increased risk of myocardial infarction (MI) [18]. Lower extremity deep vein thrombosis (DVT) is one of the more common complications following THA [19], with an incidence rate of 40–60% [20]. The development of DVT in the lower extremities can increase the risk of pulmonary embolism (PE) and other life-threatening complications as well as increase the hospital length of stay and treatment costs [19].

As outlined above, previous studies are inconclusive and present contradictory results regarding the specific complications and outcomes of TXA administration for THA. Moreover, there is a lack of a single study that examines multiple complications and patient outcomes via a large multicenter database. Considering this and the debate surrounding the efficacy of TXA, the purpose of this study is to compare complication rates and patient outcomes, at 30 days and 90 days post-procedure, between THA patients administered TXA vs. THA patients not administered TXA. This study is unique in that we will employ a large, nationally representative patient population. We hypothesize that patients administered TXA for THA will have fewer perioperative and postoperative complications compared to patients who were not administered TXA for THA.

2. Methods

2.1. Study Design and Data Source

The TriNetX Research network (https://trinetx.com, Baltimore, MD, USA) was utilized for this study. The TriNetX Research network features one of the largest repositories of data from the US, Canada, and Western Europe, encompassing inpatient, outpatient, and emergency visit data sourced from over 80 healthcare organizations (HCOs) and spanning more than 120 million patient records. Furthermore, patient data are enriched with information from over 100 commercial and government payers, including Medicare [21,22].

Patients 18 years old and above who underwent THA between 1 January 2003 and 1 January 2024 met the inclusion criteria. The data were sourced via the TriNetX database on 18 April 2024. These patients were categorized into two cohorts: (1) patients who received TXA 24 h prior to total hip arthroplasty (TXA), and (2) patients who did not receive TXA 24 h prior to total hip arthroplasty (no-TXA). The selection of patients utilized appropriate CPT, ICD-9, and ICD-10 codes. Further details on cohort construction can be found in the Supplementary Materials File.

2.2. Index Event and Outcome Analysis

The study assessed common perioperative and postoperative complications, which are further elaborated on in the Section 3. The index event was defined as the initiation of analysis for each patient, which, in this study, corresponds to the date of THA for each particular patient. The follow-up period for this study was 30 and 90 days (97% follow-up rate). Additional information on the index event, outcomes of interest, and follow-up duration is provided in the Supplementary Materials File.

2.3. Statistical Tools, Data Analysis, and Propensity Score Matching

The relative risk, supplemented by absolute risk, was used to compare the risk of complications between the exposure and comparison groups, with 95% confidence intervals provided for all relative risk calculations. The statistical tests used included Fisher's exact test and Chi-square for categorical variables, and Student's t-test for continuous variables. p values < 0.01 were considered significant.

Patients in the TXA and no-TXA cohorts were subjected to matching based on age, sex, smoking status, diabetes, and overweight/obesity status using a greedy nearest neighbor matching algorithm. Standard mean differences were analyzed to ensure balance between the cohorts after matching. The before and after matching data are presented in Table 1, and the matched characteristics can be found in the Supplementary Materials File.

Table 1. Patient demographic characteristics before match.

	Patient Demographic Characteristics (Before Match)		
	TXA (107,912)	No-TXA (72,237)	
Characteristic	n (Mean or %)	n (Mean or %)	p
Age at Index	107,912 (64.4 ± 11.1)	72,237 (63.4 ± 11.6)	<0.001
Sex			
Male	44,129 (41%)	33,476 (46%)	<0.001
Female	54,159 (50%)	37,747 (52%)	<0.001
Race and Ethnicity			
Hispanic or Latino	2501 (2%)	2754 (4%)	<0.001
Asian	1075 (1%)	537 (1%)	<0.001
Black or African American	8535 (8%)	7279 (10%)	<0.001
White	81,573 (76%)	57,752 (80%)	<0.001
Other Race	1544 (1%)	1251 (2%)	<0.001
Diagnosis			
Tobacco Use	3455 (3%)	1532 (2%)	<0.001
Diabetes Mellitus	14,865 (14%)	9260 (13%)	<0.001
BMI			
At Most 18.5 kg/m^2	1375 (1%)	1078 (1%)	<0.001
18.5–25 kg/m^2	10,068 (9%)	7148 (10%)	<0.001
25–30 kg/m^2	17,190 (16%)	12,220 (17%)	<0.001
30–35 kg/m^2	14,334 (13%)	10,546 (15%)	<0.001
35–40 kg/m^2	8309 (8%)	6098 (8%)	<0.001
At Least 40 kg/m^2	4377 (4%)	3142 (4%)	0.002

2.4. Software Used for Statistical Analysis, Validation, and Data Visualization

The TriNetX Live platform was used for data compilation. Microsoft Excel (2023) was utilized for further analysis and data visualization. The analytical procedures were verified independently by all co-authors and further confirmed by the corresponding author (SS).

2.5. Data Integrity and Ethical Considerations

All information within the TriNetX database is compliant with the Health Insurance Portability and Accountability Act (HIPAA) and contains only de-identified aggregate information [23]. As a result, this study was exempt from Institutional Review Board (IRB) approval by UT Southwestern IRB.

3. Results

3.1. Patient Demographic Data Analysis

A total of 180,149 patients were identified via the TriNetX database as having undergone THA during the specified time frame, including 107,912 patients in the TXA cohort (59.90%) and 72,237 patients in the no-TXA cohort (40.10%). The average age at the time of THA was significantly higher for the TXA patient cohort (64.4 ± 11.1) as compared to the no-TXA patient cohort (63.4 ± 11.6) ($p < 0.001$). For both the TXA and no-TXA cohorts, there was a greater proportion of female patients than male patients with 54,159 (50%) females and 44,129 (41%) males in the TXA cohort and 37,747 (52%) females and 33,476 (46%) males in the no-TXA cohort (Table 1). After propensity matching, 72,172 TXA patients and 72,172 no-TXA patients were included in the analysis. After matching, 52% of the cohort in each group were females and 46% were males ($p < 0.001$), and there were no differences in the rates of diabetes mellitus or obesity. The frequency of racial and ethnicity groups between TXA and no-TXA patients was Caucasian (82%, 80%), Black/African American (9%, 10%), Hispanic/Latino (3%, 4%), Other (2%, 2%), and Asian (1%, 1%), respectively (Table 2).

Table 2. Patient demographic characteristics after match.

Patient Demographic Characteristics (After Match)			
	TXA (72,172)	No-TXA (72,172)	
Characteristic	n (Mean or %)	n (Mean or %)	p
Age at Index	72,172 (63.4 ± 11.6)	72,172 (63.4 ± 11.6)	0.5385
Sex			
Male	33,397 (46%)	33,425 (46%)	0.883
Female	37,761 (52%)	37,733 (52%)	0.883
Race and Ethnicity			
Hispanic or Latino	1897 (3%)	2743 (4%)	<0.001
Asian	744 (1%)	535 (1%)	<0.001
Black or African American	6226 (9%)	7265 (10%)	<0.001
White	58,896 (82%)	57,712 (80%)	<0.001
Other Race	1166 (2%)	1247 (2%)	0.096
Diagnosis			
Tobacco Use	1487 (2%)	1532 (2%)	0.408
Diabetes Mellitus	9081 (13%)	9260 (13%)	0.157
BMI			
At Most 18.5 kg/m^2	951 (1%)	1055 (1%)	0.019
18.5–25 kg/m^2	6904 (10%)	7120 (10%)	0.055
25–30 kg/m^2	12,085 (17%)	12,207 (17%)	0.391
30–35 kg/m^2	10,516 (15%)	10,537 (15%)	0.876
35–40 kg/m^2	6002 (8%)	6096 (8%)	0.372
At Least 40 kg/m^2	3075 (4%)	3142 (4%)	0.385

3.2. Analysis of Patient Complications

Thirty-Day Follow-Up:

At 30 days following THA, TXA patients had a reduced risk of transfusion (risk ratio (RR): 0.412; 95% confidence interval (CI): 0.374, 0.453), reduced risk of DVT (RR: 0.856; CI: 0.768, 0.953), reduced risk of periprosthetic joint infection (RR: 0.808; CI: 0.710, 0.920), but a higher rate of periprosthetic fracture (RR: 1.234; CI: 1.065, 1.429) compared to patients who did not receive TXA. There were no significant differences between the two groups regarding the rates of MI, PE, hematoma formation, acute renal failure, wound dehiscence, pneumonia, deep or superficial surgical site infection (SSI), and periprosthetic dislocation (Table 3).

Table 3. Table of risk ratios (30-day follow-up—matched).

Measure	TXA (n)	No-TXA (n)	TXA Proportion	No-TXA Proportion	Risk Ratio	95% CI	p
Transfusion	593	1440	0.8%	2.0%	0.412	(0.374, 0.453)	<0.001
Myocardial Infarction	271	267	0.4%	0.4%	1.015	(0.857, 1.201)	0.863
Pulmonary Embolism	373	412	0.5%	0.6%	0.905	(0.787, 1.041)	0.163
Deep Vein Thrombosis (Lower Extremity)	605	707	0.8%	1.0%	0.856	(0.768, 0.953)	0.005
Hematoma	39	34	0.1%	0.0%	1.147	(0.724, 1.817)	0.558
Periprosthetic Joint Infection	409	506	0.6%	0.7%	0.808	(0.710, 0.920)	0.001
Acute Renal Failure	939	1018	1.3%	1.4%	0.922	(0.845, 1.007)	0.072
Acute Posthemorrhagic Anemia	3796	3129	5.3%	4.3%	1.213	(1.158, 1.271)	<0.001
Wound Dehiscence	312	291	0.4%	0.4%	1.072	(0.914, 1.257)	0.391
Pneumonia	351	404	0.5%	0.6%	0.869	(0.753, 1.002)	0.053
Deep SSI	26	18	0.0%	0.0%	1.444	(0.792, 2.634)	0.228
Superficial SSI	107	55	0.1%	0.1%	1.945	(1.406, 2.693)	<0.001
Periprosthetic Mechanical Complication	75	99	0.1%	0.1%	0.758	(0.561, 1.022)	0.069
Periprosthetic Dislocation	330	357	0.5%	0.5%	0.924	(0.796, 1.073)	0.302
Periprosthetic Fracture	396	321	0.5%	0.4%	1.234	(1.065, 1.429)	0.005
Subgroup Analysis							
Myocardial Infarction (Previous Stent/CABG vs. No Previous Stent/CABG)	33	21	4.3%	2.7%	1.571	(0.918, 2.691)	0.097

Ninety-Day Follow-Up:

At 90 days following THA, TXA patients had a reduced risk of transfusion (RR: 0.446; CI: 0.408, 0.487), DVT (RR: 0.847; CI: 0.776, 0.924), and periprosthetic joint infection (RR: 0.894; CI: 0.815, 0.982) compared to patients who did not receive TXA. Patients who received TXA had higher rates of periprosthetic fracture (RR: 1.219; CI: 1.088, 1.365), acute postoperative anemia (RR: 1.222; CI: 1.171, 1.276), deep SSI (RR: 1.706; CI: 1.117, 2.605), and superficial SSI (RR: 1.950; CI: 1.567, 2.428) compared to patients who did not receive TXA. There were no significant differences between the two groups at 90 days regarding the rates of MI, hematoma formation, acute renal failure, pneumonia, wound dehiscence, and prosthetic-related dislocations and mechanical complications (Table 4).

Table 4. Table of risk ratios (90-day follow-up—matched).

Measure	TXA (N)	No-TXA (n)	TXA Proportion	No-TXA Proportion	Risk Ratio	95% CI	p
Transfusion	713	1599	1.0%	2.2%	0.446	(0.408, 0.487)	<0.001
Myocardial Infarction	385	402	0.5%	0.6%	0.958	(0.833, 1.101)	0.543
Pulmonary Embolism	565	634	0.8%	0.9%	0.891	(0.796, 0.998)	0.045
Deep Vein Thrombosis (Lower Extremity)	920	1086	1.3%	1.5%	0.847	(0.776, 0.924)	<0.001
Hematoma	58	48	0.1%	0.1%	1.208	(0.824, 1.771)	0.331
Periprosthetic Joint Infection	830	928	1.2%	1.3%	0.894	(0.815, 0.982)	0.019
Acute Renal Failure	1298	1328	1.8%	1.8%	0.977	(0.906, 1.054)	0.555

Table 4. *Cont.*

Measure	Table of Risk Ratios—90-Day F/U (Matched)						
	TXA (N)	No-TXA (*n*)	TXA Proportion	No-TXA Proportion	Risk Ratio	95% CI	*p*
Acute Posthemorrhagic Anemia	4415	3612	6.1%	5.0%	1.222	(1.171, 1.276)	<0.001
Wound Dehiscence	626	552	0.9%	0.8%	1.134	(1.012, 1.271)	0.030
Pneumonia	568	614	0.8%	0.9%	0.925	(0.826, 1.036)	0.179
Deep SSI	58	34	0.1%	0.0%	1.706	(1.117, 2.605)	0.012
Superficial SSI	236	121	0.3%	0.2%	1.950	(1.567, 2.428)	<0.001
Periprosthetic Mechanical Complication	191	196	0.3%	0.3%	0.974	(0.799, 1.189)	0.799
Periprosthetic Dislocation	603	647	0.8%	0.9%	0.932	(0.835, 1.041)	0.211
Periprosthetic Fracture	658	540	0.9%	0.7%	1.219	(1.088, 1.365)	0.001
Subgroup Analysis							
Myocardial Infarction (Previous Stent/CABG vs. No Previous Stent/CABG)	46	35	5.9%	4.5%	1.314	(0.857, 2.017)	0.209

4. Discussion

The utilization of THA continues to increase, especially with the increasing average patient age and consequent higher prevalence of degenerative hip diseases [4,24]. The indications for the surgical administration of TXA, as a cost-effective measure to minimize blood loss, are also continuing to expand [25,26]. However, the thrombotic and life-threatening cardiovascular complications associated with TXA administration has limited widespread employment of TXA [3,17,18,27].

Patients in the no-TXA cohort had a greater need for blood transfusions at both the 30-day and 90-day follow-ups compared to the patients in the TXA cohort. Given that TXA serves an antifibrinolytic role and minimizes blood loss [13,28,29], this finding is consistent with our hypothesis. Our analysis is supported by a study by Stoicea et al. which found that TXA, via both intravenous and intra-articular forms, reduced decreases in both postoperative hemoglobin and hematocrit following primary posterior and revision THA, indicating the efficacy of TXA in minimizing blood loss and transfusion [3]. Other studies and reviews also align with our finding that TXA promotes hemostasis and reduces intraoperative blood loss in orthopedic procedures [2,12,30].

Patients in the TXA cohort had a significantly reduced risk of DVT and need for transfusion compared to patients in the no-TXA cohort at both 30 and 90 days. These results are congruent with most of the previous orthopedic literature, apart from the findings of TXA reduction in the rates of DVT. Two separate meta-analyses of randomized controlled trials, investigating the efficacy and safety of TXA in orthopedic lower limb surgeries, reported that TXA did not increase the risk of venous thromboembolism, and it reduced blood loss, transfusion requirements, and length of hospital stay without any additional thromboembolic risk [14,31]. Other studies reported similar findings that the use of high-dose TXA does not influence the prevalence of MI, DVT, and PE [3,32–34]. Although some studies have found correlations between TXA and MI [18,27,34], these studies primarily studied patients at high-risk for cardiovascular disease. We did not observe any difference in the rate of postoperative MI between the two groups.

An interesting observation was that patients who received TXA had higher rates of superficial SSI at 30 days and higher rates of both superficial and deep infection as well as prosthetic fracture at 90 days. These findings are not concordant with the current consensus that TXA is not known to be associated with increasing rates of SSI. A meta-analysis reviewed 31 articles and concluded that the intravenous administration of TXA reduces the incidence of overall infection, including SSI, in patients undergoing both THA and TKA [35]. One hypothesized mechanism for this decrease in infection rates is TXA-associated changes in immune marker expression on immune cell subsets and decreased levels of proinflammatory cytokines, both of which are correlated with a lower rate of postoperative infection [36]. Moreover, blood transfusion is a known risk for prosthetic joint infection [35], but the TXA cohort had decreased rates of blood transfusion. We do not have a good explanation for this finding since the rate of postoperative hematoma formation was not different between the two groups. Kramer et al. found that there is no added risk for wound healing problems or SSI attributable to preoperative TXA in spine surgeries [37]. This discrepancy can be explained by patient demographics: a large proportion of the patients undergoing THA are geriatric [4], a patient population that presents with comorbidities and at higher risk for orthopedic and non-orthopedic complications, such as SSI and periprosthetic fracture [38]. The lack of difference in hematoma complications between TXA and no-TXA groups are in congruence with the previous literature given that TXA mechanistically works to prevent hematomas [39].

Patients undergoing THA who were given preoperative TXA had lower rates of periprosthetic joint infection at the 30- and 90-day follow-ups compared to patients who did not receive preoperative TXA. These findings are consistent with the previous literature. Yazdi et al. studied TXA in primary joint arthroplasty and reported that TXA helps to reduce the rate of periprosthetic joint infection. The authors proposed that a reduction in bleeding and a lower need for allogenic blood transfusion may be responsible for the lower incidence of infection [40]. Another study, upon adjusting for multiple patient characteristics and surgical factors, independently associated TXA with a reduced risk of subsequent acute periprosthetic joint infection [41]. Additionally, other researchers concluded that TXA has inhibitory effects against implant infections by reducing surgical site bleeding and associated biofilm formation [42]. Regarding acute renal failure, although there is research in the literature suggesting a potential renal effect of TXA and discouraging administration of TXA to patients with kidney dysfunction [29], we found no significant differences in kidney failure between TXA and no-TXA cohorts.

A statistically significant difference in wound dehiscence was not observed at the 30-day follow-up. Several studies have reported that TXA did not add risk to wound healing complications in orthopedic procedures [37,43]. Our study agrees with the literature regarding the negligible effect of TXA on wound healing complications.

Our study's inherent limitations stem from its retrospective nature and the fact that patient data were sourced from EHRs which are susceptible to errors in coding and documentation. The TriNetX database is a voluntary program, and selection bias may be present due to overrepresentation by large, academic research institutions. TriNetX provides temporality on a day-to-day level, and the route of administration and dosage information was lacking, and therefore, it was excluded from the analysis. Hence, TriNetX cannot provide more specific timing information. Furthermore, the data may not be representative of the entire global population. We could not adjust our outcomes of interest after THA for socioeconomic variables such health insurance, education level, and income, and we acknowledge that these variables are important to consider, particularly in any study that outcomes after surgery.

Since the patient data were derived from a diverse range of medical practices and locations across the US, Western Europe, and Canada, there were likely variations in surgical equipment, surgical techniques, reporting of medical and surgical complications, and post-operative patient protocol. For example, the specific type of periprosthetic joint infection and its exact treatment course is not known for each individual patient. Moreover, retrospective studies are reliant on the medical personnel to record patient data. Any inaccuracies in data entry or reporting may have influenced the results and analysis of our study. However, the size of our patient cohorts mitigates these risks and enhances the predictive power of the study, allowing for a more accurate estimate of rare complications. Additionally, all complications of interest were decided upon prior to collecting data, which solidifies the reliability of the study. Regarding biases, because none of the study's

Table 4. Cont.

Measure	TXA (N)	No-TXA (n)	TXA Proportion	No-TXA Proportion	Risk Ratio	95% CI	p
		Table of Risk Ratios—90-Day F/U (Matched)					
Acute Posthemorrhagic Anemia	4415	3612	6.1%	5.0%	1.222	(1.171, 1.276)	<0.001
Wound Dehiscence	626	552	0.9%	0.8%	1.134	(1.012, 1.271)	0.030
Pneumonia	568	614	0.8%	0.9%	0.925	(0.826, 1.036)	0.179
Deep SSI	58	34	0.1%	0.0%	1.706	(1.117, 2.605)	0.012
Superficial SSI	236	121	0.3%	0.2%	1.950	(1.567, 2.428)	<0.001
Periprosthetic Mechanical Complication	191	196	0.3%	0.3%	0.974	(0.799, 1.189)	0.799
Periprosthetic Dislocation	603	647	0.8%	0.9%	0.932	(0.835, 1.041)	0.211
Periprosthetic Fracture	658	540	0.9%	0.7%	1.219	(1.088, 1.365)	0.001
Subgroup Analysis							
Myocardial Infarction (Previous Stent/CABG vs. No Previous Stent/CABG)	46	35	5.9%	4.5%	1.314	(0.857, 2.017)	0.209

4. Discussion

The utilization of THA continues to increase, especially with the increasing average patient age and consequent higher prevalence of degenerative hip diseases [4,24]. The indications for the surgical administration of TXA, as a cost-effective measure to minimize blood loss, are also continuing to expand [25,26]. However, the thrombotic and life-threatening cardiovascular complications associated with TXA administration has limited widespread employment of TXA [3,17,18,27].

Patients in the no-TXA cohort had a greater need for blood transfusions at both the 30-day and 90-day follow-ups compared to the patients in the TXA cohort. Given that TXA serves an antifibrinolytic role and minimizes blood loss [13,28,29], this finding is consistent with our hypothesis. Our analysis is supported by a study by Stoicea et al. which found that TXA, via both intravenous and intra-articular forms, reduced decreases in both postoperative hemoglobin and hematocrit following primary posterior and revision THA, indicating the efficacy of TXA in minimizing blood loss and transfusion [3]. Other studies and reviews also align with our finding that TXA promotes hemostasis and reduces intraoperative blood loss in orthopedic procedures [2,12,30].

Patients in the TXA cohort had a significantly reduced risk of DVT and need for transfusion compared to patients in the no-TXA cohort at both 30 and 90 days. These results are congruent with most of the previous orthopedic literature, apart from the findings of TXA reduction in the rates of DVT. Two separate meta-analyses of randomized controlled trials, investigating the efficacy and safety of TXA in orthopedic lower limb surgeries, reported that TXA did not increase the risk of venous thromboembolism, and it reduced blood loss, transfusion requirements, and length of hospital stay without any additional thromboembolic risk [14,31]. Other studies reported similar findings that the use of high-dose TXA does not influence the prevalence of MI, DVT, and PE [3,32–34]. Although some studies have found correlations between TXA and MI [18,27,34], these studies primarily studied patients at high-risk for cardiovascular disease. We did not observe any difference in the rate of postoperative MI between the two groups.

An interesting observation was that patients who received TXA had higher rates of superficial SSI at 30 days and higher rates of both superficial and deep infection as well as prosthetic fracture at 90 days. These findings are not concordant with the current consensus that TXA is not known to be associated with increasing rates of SSI. A meta-analysis reviewed 31 articles and concluded that the intravenous administration of TXA reduces the incidence of overall infection, including SSI, in patients undergoing both THA and TKA [35]. One hypothesized mechanism for this decrease in infection rates is TXA-associated changes in immune marker expression on immune cell subsets and decreased levels of proinflammatory cytokines, both of which are correlated with a lower rate of postoperative infection [36]. Moreover, blood transfusion is a known risk for prosthetic joint infection [35], but the TXA cohort had decreased rates of blood transfusion. We do not have a good explanation for this finding since the rate of postoperative hematoma formation was not different between the two groups. Kramer et al. found that there is no added risk for wound healing problems or SSI attributable to preoperative TXA in spine surgeries [37]. This discrepancy can be explained by patient demographics: a large proportion of the patients undergoing THA are geriatric [4], a patient population that presents with comorbidities and at higher risk for orthopedic and non-orthopedic complications, such as SSI and periprosthetic fracture [38]. The lack of difference in hematoma complications between TXA and no-TXA groups are in congruence with the previous literature given that TXA mechanistically works to prevent hematomas [39].

Patients undergoing THA who were given preoperative TXA had lower rates of periprosthetic joint infection at the 30- and 90-day follow-ups compared to patients who did not receive preoperative TXA. These findings are consistent with the previous literature. Yazdi et al. studied TXA in primary joint arthroplasty and reported that TXA helps to reduce the rate of periprosthetic joint infection. The authors proposed that a reduction in bleeding and a lower need for allogenic blood transfusion may be responsible for the lower incidence of infection [40]. Another study, upon adjusting for multiple patient characteristics and surgical factors, independently associated TXA with a reduced risk of subsequent acute periprosthetic joint infection [41]. Additionally, other researchers concluded that TXA has inhibitory effects against implant infections by reducing surgical site bleeding and associated biofilm formation [42]. Regarding acute renal failure, although there is research in the literature suggesting a potential renal effect of TXA and discouraging administration of TXA to patients with kidney dysfunction [29], we found no significant differences in kidney failure between TXA and no-TXA cohorts.

A statistically significant difference in wound dehiscence was not observed at the 30-day follow-up. Several studies have reported that TXA did not add risk to wound healing complications in orthopedic procedures [37,43]. Our study agrees with the literature regarding the negligible effect of TXA on wound healing complications.

Our study's inherent limitations stem from its retrospective nature and the fact that patient data were sourced from EHRs which are susceptible to errors in coding and documentation. The TriNetX database is a voluntary program, and selection bias may be present due to overrepresentation by large, academic research institutions. TriNetX provides temporality on a day-to-day level, and the route of administration and dosage information was lacking, and therefore, it was excluded from the analysis. Hence, TriNetX cannot provide more specific timing information. Furthermore, the data may not be representative of the entire global population. We could not adjust our outcomes of interest after THA for socioeconomic variables such health insurance, education level, and income, and we acknowledge that these variables are important to consider, particularly in any study that outcomes after surgery.

Since the patient data were derived from a diverse range of medical practices and locations across the US, Western Europe, and Canada, there were likely variations in surgical equipment, surgical techniques, reporting of medical and surgical complications, and post-operative patient protocol. For example, the specific type of periprosthetic joint infection and its exact treatment course is not known for each individual patient. Moreover, retrospective studies are reliant on the medical personnel to record patient data. Any inaccuracies in data entry or reporting may have influenced the results and analysis of our study. However, the size of our patient cohorts mitigates these risks and enhances the predictive power of the study, allowing for a more accurate estimate of rare complications. Additionally, all complications of interest were decided upon prior to collecting data, which solidifies the reliability of the study. Regarding biases, because none of the study's authors participated in the actual surgical procedures and patients were de-identified, the possibility of bias was reduced, further enhancing the reliability of our findings.

Despite the limitations described, a particular strength of this study is the ability to analyze a large, matched cohort of patients who underwent THA, incorporating important demographic factors and comorbidities. To the best of our knowledge, this is the largest known patient cohort to be used in comparing THA patient outcomes in patients who received or did not receive preoperative TXA. Additionally, this study is strengthened by its use of propensity score matching, a validated observational cohort comparison technique, which helps remove any confounding bias [44]. Propensity score matching allows for factors such as age, sex, obesity status, and tobacco use from confounding the result outputs. We recognize that 90 days is a relatively short period of follow-up, but this should be adequate to address the potential complications of TXA following THA. Given that many hospital metrics are based on 90-day mortality, longer follow-up periods may also alter measurements and change the significance of the findings.

5. Conclusions

At 30 days following THA, TXA patients had a reduced risk of transfusion, reduced risk of DVT, reduced risk of prosthetic joint infection, but a higher rate of periprosthetic fracture compared to patients who did not receive TXA. At 90 days following THA, TXA patients had a reduced risk of transfusion, lower extremity DVT, and prosthetic joint infection compared to patients who did not receive TXA. At 90 days following THA, patients who received TXA had higher rates of postoperative anemia, deep SSI, and superficial SSI compared to patients who did not receive TXA. No significant differences in the rates of postoperative MI were observed between the two groups at either the 30- or 90-day follow-up following THA. Future studies should examine the complications of TXA with other arthroplasty procedures and aim for long-term follow-up and with a large, representative patient population.

Supplementary Materials: The following supporting information can be downloaded at: https://www.mdpi.com/article/10.3390/jcm13164920/s1. Supplementary Materials File.

Author Contributions: A.T.: validation, writing—original draft, writing—review and editing, project administration; M.M.M.: data processing, data curation, validation, writing—review and editing, visualization; T.L.R.: validation, writing—reviewing and editing, V.M.: validation, writing—reviewing and editing; D.K.W.: validation, writing—reviewing and editing; S.N.S.: conceptualization, methodology, software, writing—review and editing, supervision, project administration. All work for this manuscript was performed on the premises of University of Texas Southwestern Medical School (5323 Harry Hines Blvd, Dallas, TX, USA, 75390). All authors have read and agreed to the published version of the manuscript.

Funding: This research received no external funding.

Institutional Review Board Statement: This study was exempt from IRB approval since the data were de-identified and publicly available.

Informed Consent Statement: This retrospective study is exempt from informed consent. The data reviewed represent a secondary analysis of existing data, do not involve intervention or interaction with human subjects, and are de-identified per the de-identification standard defined in Section §164.514(a) of the HIPAA Privacy Rule. The process by which the data are de-identified is attested to through a formal determination by a qualified expert as defined in Section §164.514(b)(1) of the HIPAA Privacy Rule. This formal determination by a qualified expert was refreshed on December 2020.

Data Availability Statement: The data that support the findings of this study are available from TriNetX. Restrictions apply to the availability of these data, which were used under license for this study. Data are available from https://trinetx.com with the permission from TriNetX.

Conflicts of Interest: All authors certify that they have no affiliations with or involvement in any organization or entity with any financial interests or non-financial interests in the subject matter or materials discussed in this manuscript.

References

1. Melvin, J.S.; Stryker, L.S.; Sierra, R.J. Tranexamic Acid in Hip and Knee Arthroplasty. *J. Am. Acad. Orthop. Surg.* **2015**, *23*, 732–740. [CrossRef] [PubMed]
2. Goldstein, M.; Feldmann, C.; Wulf, H.; Wiesmann, T. Tranexamic Acid Prophylaxis in Hip and Knee Joint Replacement. *Dtsch. Arztebl. Int.* **2017**, *114*, 824–830. [CrossRef]
3. Stoicea, N.; Moran, K.; Mahmoud, A.R.; Glassman, A.; Ellis, T.; Ryan, J.; Granger, J.; Joseph, N.; Salon, N.; Ackermann, W.; et al. Tranexamic acid use during total hip arthroplasty: A single center retrospective analysis. *Medicine* **2018**, *97*, e10720. [CrossRef] [PubMed]
4. Patel, I.; Nham, F.; Zalikha, A.K.; El-Othmani, M.M. Epidemiology of total hip arthroplasty: Demographics, comorbidities and outcomes. *Arthroplasty* **2023**, *5*, 2. [CrossRef] [PubMed]
5. Bric, J.D.; Miley, E.N.; Parvataneni, H.K.; Pulido, L.; Prieto, H.A.; Gray, C.F.; Deen, J.T. Outpatient total hip and knee arthroplasty—Patient expectations versus experience. *J. Orthop.* **2024**, *51*, 109–115. [CrossRef] [PubMed]
6. Dhaliwal, A.S.; Akhtar, M.; Razick, D.I.; Afzali, A.; Wilson, E.; Nedopil, A.J. Current Surgical Techniques in the Treatment of Adult Developmental Dysplasia of the Hip. *J. Pers. Med.* **2023**, *13*, 942. [CrossRef]
7. Li, J.; Zhu, H.; Liao, R. Enhanced recovery after surgery (ERAS) pathway for primary hip and knee arthroplasty: Study protocol for a randomized controlled trial. *Trials* **2019**, *20*, 599. [CrossRef]
8. Krumme, J.W.; Bonanni, S.; Patel, N.K.; Golladay, G.J. Technical Considerations and Avoiding Complications in Total Hip Arthroplasty. *J. Am. Acad. Orthop. Surg. Glob. Res. Rev.* **2022**, *6*, e22.00234. [CrossRef]
9. Sloan, M.; Premkumar, A.; Sheth, N.P. Projected Volume of Primary Total Joint Arthroplasty in the U.S., 2014 to 2030. *J. Bone Joint Surg. Am.* **2018**, *100*, 1455–1460. [CrossRef]
10. Kelmer, G.; Stone, A.H.; Turcotte, J.; King, P.J. Reasons for Revision: Primary Total Hip Arthroplasty Mechanisms of Failure. *J. Am. Acad. Orthop. Surg.* **2021**, *29*, 78–87. [CrossRef]
11. Erivan, R.; Villatte, G.; Ollivier, M.; Paprosky, W.G. Painful Hip Arthroplasty: What Should We Find? Diagnostic Approach and Results. *J. Arthroplast.* **2019**, *34*, 1802–1807. [CrossRef]
12. Cai, L.; Chen, L.; Zhao, C.; Wang, Q.; Kang, P. Influencing factors of hidden blood loss after primary total hip arthroplasty through the posterior approach: A retrospective study. *BMC Musculoskelet. Disord.* **2023**, *24*, 582. [CrossRef]
13. Vrontis, K.; Tsinaslanidis, G.; Drosos, G.I.; Tzatzairis, T. Perioperative Blood Management Strategies for Patients Undergoing Total Hip Arthroplasty: Where Do We Currently Stand on This Matter? *Arch. Bone Jt. Surg.* **2020**, *8*, 646–655. [CrossRef]
14. Zhu, J.; Zhu, Y.; Lei, P.; Zeng, M.; Su, W.; Hu, Y. Efficacy and safety of tranexamic acid in total hip replacement: A PRISMA-compliant meta-analysis of 25 randomized controlled trials. *Medicine* **2017**, *96*, e9552. [CrossRef] [PubMed]
15. Fillingham, Y.A.; Ramkumar, D.B.; Jevsevar, D.S.; Yates, A.J.; Shores, P.; Mullen, K.; Bini, S.A.; Clarke, H.D.; Schemitsch, E.; Johnson, R.L.; et al. The Efficacy of Tranexamic Acid in Total Hip Arthroplasty: A Network Meta-analysis. *J. Arthroplasty* **2018**, *33*, 3083–3089.e3084. [CrossRef]
16. Ghorbani, M.; Sadrian, S.H.; Ghaderpanah, R.; Neitzke, C.C.; Chalmers, B.P.; Esmaeilian, S.; Rahmanipour, E.; Parsa, A. Tranexamic acid in total hip arthroplasty: An umbrella review on efficacy and safety. *J. Orthop.* **2024**, *54*, 90–102. [CrossRef] [PubMed]
17. Myers, S.P.; Kutcher, M.E.; Rosengart, M.R.; Sperry, J.L.; Peitzman, A.B.; Brown, J.B.; Neal, M.D. Tranexamic acid administration is associated with an increased risk of posttraumatic venous thromboembolism. *J. Trauma Acute Care Surg.* **2019**, *86*, 20–27. [CrossRef] [PubMed]
18. Yao, Y.T.; Yuan, X.; Shao, K. Acute Myocardial Infarction After Tranexamic Acid: Review of Published Case Reports. *Chin. Med. Sci. J.* **2020**, *35*, 65–70. [CrossRef]
19. Yu, X.; Wu, Y.; Ning, R. The deep vein thrombosis of lower limb after total hip arthroplasty: What should we care. *BMC Musculoskelet Disord.* **2021**, *22*, 547. [CrossRef]
20. Wainwright, T.W.; Gill, M.; McDonald, D.A.; Middleton, R.G.; Reed, M.; Sahota, O.; Yates, P.; Ljungqvist, O. Consensus statement for perioperative care in total hip replacement and total knee replacement surgery: Enhanced Recovery After Surgery (ERAS((R))) Society recommendations. *Acta. Orthop.* **2020**, *91*, 3–19. [CrossRef]
21. Palchuk, M.B.; London, J.W.; Perez-Rey, D.; Drebert, Z.J.; Winer-Jones, J.P.; Thompson, C.N.; Esposito, J.; Claerhout, B. A global federated real-world data and analytics platform for research. *JAMIA Open* **2023**, *6*, ooad035. [CrossRef]
22. TriNetX. Real World Data—Linked. Available online: https://trinetx.com/real-world-data/linked/ (accessed on 28 April 2024).
23. TriNetX. Publication Guidelines. Available online: https://trinetx.com/real-world-resources/publications/trinetx-publication-guidelines/ (accessed on 28 April 2024).
24. Delsmann, M.M.; Strahl, A.; Muhlenfeld, M.; Jandl, N.M.; Beil, F.T.; Ries, C.; Rolvien, T. High prevalence and undertreatment of osteoporosis in elderly patients undergoing total hip arthroplasty. *Osteoporos. Int.* **2021**, *32*, 1661–1668. [CrossRef]
25. Cartagena-Reyes, M.A.; Silva-Aponte, J.A.; Nazario-Ferrer, G.I.; Benes, G.A.; Choudhary, A.; Raad, M.; Frank, S.M.; Musharbash, F.N.; Jain, A. The cost-utility of intraoperative tranexamic acid in adult spinal deformity patients undergoing long posterior spinal fusion. *Spine Deform.* **2024**, *12*, 587–593. [CrossRef]
26. Sukeik, M.; Alshryda, S.; Haddad, F.S.; Mason, J.M. Systematic review and meta-analysis of the use of tranexamic acid in total hip replacement. *J. Bone Joint Surg. Br.* **2011**, *93*, 39–46. [CrossRef] [PubMed]

27. Kaptein, Y.E. Acute ST-elevation myocardial infarction due to in-stent thrombosis after administering tranexamic acid in a high cardiac risk patient. *BMJ Case Rep.* **2019**, *12*, e227957. [CrossRef] [PubMed]
28. Meng, Y.; Li, Z.; Gong, K.; An, X.; Dong, J.; Tang, P. Tranexamic acid reduces intraoperative occult blood loss and tourniquet time in obese knee osteoarthritis patients undergoing total knee arthroplasty: A prospective cohort study. *Ther. Clin. Risk Manag.* **2018**, *14*, 675–683. [CrossRef]
29. Pabinger, I.; Fries, D.; Schochl, H.; Streif, W.; Toller, W. Tranexamic acid for treatment and prophylaxis of bleeding and hyperfibrinolysis. *Wien. Klin. Wochenschr* **2017**, *129*, 303–316. [CrossRef] [PubMed]
30. Haratian, A.; Shelby, T.; Hasan, L.K.; Bolia, I.K.; Weber, A.E.; Petrigliano, F.A. Utilization of Tranexamic Acid in Surgical Orthopaedic Practice: Indications and Current Considerations. *Orthop. Res. Rev.* **2021**, *13*, 187–199. [CrossRef] [PubMed]
31. Reale, D.; Andriolo, L.; Gursoy, S.; Bozkurt, M.; Filardo, G.; Zaffagnini, S. Complications of Tranexamic Acid in Orthopedic Lower Limb Surgery: A Meta-Analysis of Randomized Controlled Trials. *Biomed. Res. Int.* **2021**, *2021*, 6961540. [CrossRef]
32. Nishihara, S.; Hamada, M. Does tranexamic acid alter the risk of thromboembolism after total hip arthroplasty in the absence of routine chemical thromboprophylaxis? *Bone Joint J.* **2015**, *97-B*, 458–462. [CrossRef] [PubMed]
33. Ollivier, J.E.; Van Driessche, S.; Billuart, F.; Beldame, J.; Matsoukis, J. Tranexamic acid and total hip arthroplasty: Optimizing the administration method. *Ann. Transl. Med.* **2016**, *4*, 530. [CrossRef]
34. Wang, E.; Wang, Y.; Li, Y.; Hu, S.; Yuan, S. Tranexamic acid is associated with improved hemostasis in elderly patients undergoing coronary-artery surgeries in a retrospective cohort study. *Front Surg.* **2023**, *10*, 1117974. [CrossRef] [PubMed]
35. Imanishi, K.; Kobayashi, N.; Kamono, E.; Yukizawa, Y.; Takagawa, S.; Choe, H.; Kumagai, K.; Inaba, Y. Tranexamic acid administration for the prevention of periprosthetic joint infection and surgical site infection: A systematic review and meta-analysis. *Arch. Orthop. Trauma Surg.* **2023**, *143*, 6883–6899. [CrossRef]
36. Draxler, D.F.; Yep, K.; Hanafi, G.; Winton, A.; Daglas, M.; Ho, H.; Sashindranath, M.; Wutzlhofer, L.M.; Forbes, A.; Goncalves, I.; et al. Tranexamic acid modulates the immune response and reduces postsurgical infection rates. *Blood Adv.* **2019**, *3*, 1598–1609. [CrossRef]
37. Kramer, M.; Drexler, M.; Herman, A.; Kalimian, T.; Klassov, Y.; Nasser, L.A. Use of Intraoperative Tranexamic Acid and Wound Complications in Spine Surgery: A Retrospective Cohort Study. *Asian Spine J.* **2020**, *14*, 639–646. [CrossRef] [PubMed]
38. Anderson, P.M.; Vollmann, P.; Weissenberger, M.; Rudert, M. Total hip arthroplasty in geriatric patients—A single-center experience. *SICOT-J* **2022**, *8*, 12. [CrossRef] [PubMed]
39. Yan, Z.; Chen, S.; Xue, T.; Wu, X.; Song, Z.; Wang, Z.; Chen, Z.; Wang, Z. The Function of Tranexamic Acid to Prevent Hematoma Expansion After Intracerebral Hemorrhage: A Systematic Review and Meta-Analysis from Randomized Controlled Trials. *Front. Neurol.* **2021**, *12*, 710568. [CrossRef]
40. Yazdi, H.; Klement, M.R.; Hammad, M.; Inoue, D.; Xu, C.; Goswami, K.; Parvizi, J. Tranexamic Acid Is Associated With Reduced Periprosthetic Joint Infection After Primary Total Joint Arthroplasty. *J. Arthroplasty* **2020**, *35*, 840–844. [CrossRef]
41. Klement, M.R.; Padua, F.G.; Li, W.T.; Detweiler, M.; Parvizi, J. Tranexamic Acid Reduces the Rate of Periprosthetic Joint Infection After Aseptic Revision Arthroplasty. *J. Bone Joint Surg. Am.* **2020**, *102*, 1344–1350. [CrossRef] [PubMed]
42. Wang, J.; Zhang, Z.; Li, J.; Huang, B.; Jiang, Z.; Pan, Y.; He, T.; Hu, Y.; Wang, L. Tranexamic acid protects against implant-associated infection by reducing biofilm formation. *Sci. Rep.* **2022**, *12*, 4840. [CrossRef]
43. Gupta, A.; Singh, M.; Raina, P.; Singh, S.; Ahmad, S.; Imran, S.; Sharma, R.; Malhotra, S. Post-Surgical Wound Care In Orthopedics: Role of Tranexamic Acid. *J. Evol. Med. Dent. Sci.* **2015**, *4*, 5716–5720. [CrossRef]
44. Kane, L.T.; Fang, T.; Galetta, M.S.; Goyal, D.K.C.; Nicholson, K.J.; Kepler, C.K.; Vaccaro, A.R.; Schroeder, G.D. Propensity Score Matching: A Statistical Method. *Clin. Spine Surg.* **2020**, *33*, 120–122. [CrossRef] [PubMed]

Disclaimer/Publisher's Note: The statements, opinions and data contained in all publications are solely those of the individual author(s) and contributor(s) and not of MDPI and/or the editor(s). MDPI and/or the editor(s) disclaim responsibility for any injury to people or property resulting from any ideas, methods, instructions or products referred to in the content.

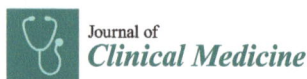

Systematic Review

The Use of Highly Porous 3-D-Printed Titanium Acetabular Cups in Revision Total Hip Arthroplasty: A Systematic Review and Meta-Analysis

Peter Richard Almeida [1,*], Gavin J. Macpherson [1,2], Philip Simpson [1,2], Paul Gaston [1,2] and Nick D. Clement [1,2,*]

1. Edinburgh Orthopaedics, Royal Infirmary of Edinburgh, Edinburgh EH16 4SA, UK
2. Department of Orthopaedics and Trauma, University of Edinburgh, Edinburgh EH8 9YL, UK
* Correspondence: rich.almeida11@gmail.com (P.R.A.); nickclement@doctors.org.uk (N.D.C.)

Abstract: Background/Objectives: As the rate of revision total hip arthroplasty (THA) has risen, there has been a drive to improve the technology in the manufacturing of the implants used. One recent advance has been 3-D printing of trabecular titanium implants to improve implant stability and osteointegration. The aim of this study was to review the clinical and radiological outcomes of these acetabular implants in revision THA. **Methods**: A manual search of the databases of the US National Library of medicine (PubMed/MEDLINE), Embase, and the Cochrane library was performed. The following keywords of "revision total hip arthroplasty" AND "acetabulum" AND "titanium" AND "porous" were utilised. **Results**: In total, 106 abstracts were identified during manual search of databases. In total, 11 studies reporting 4 different implants, with a total of 597 operated joints in 585 patients were included in this review. There were 349 (59.7%) female patients, and the mean age per study ranged from 56.0 to 78.4 years. The all-cause survival rate was 95.52% (95% CI: 92.37–97.96) at a mean follow up of 3.8 years (95% CI: 2.6–5.1). The 40 cases that required re-operation included 17 (2.8%) for infection, 14 (2.3%) instability, 2 (0.3%) for shell migration and 5 (0.8%) for aseptic loosening. The most commonly used patient reported outcome measure was the Harris Hip Score with the mean post-operative score of 86.7 (95% CI: 84.3–89.1). **Conclusions**: Trabecular titanium acetabular implants, when used in revision THA, resulted in excellent short- to mid-term outcomes with improved hip specific outcomes and a survivorship of 95.52% over the reported follow-up period. Future prospective studies evaluating long term outcomes are needed to make comparisons between more established solutions used in revision THA.

Keywords: revision total hip arthroplasty; acetabulum; titanium; additive manufacturing

1. Introduction

Over one million total hip arthroplasty (THA) procedures are performed annually worldwide, and the procedure is regarded as one of the most successful orthopaedic interventions [1,2]. THA is a cost-effective treatment for end-stage osteoarthritis of the hip with the majority of patients enjoying improvement in pain, hip function and health related quality of life within the first year after surgery [3]. The annual number of THAs performed is predicted to increase by 176% by the year 2040 and 659% by the year 2060 in the United States of America alone [4–6]. More than half of primary THA will survive past 25 years, leaving many requiring revisions during the lifetime of the recipient [7]. In keeping with rising numbers of primary THA there is a parallel increase in the number of revision THAs [3,8]. In the United States alone, revision THA grew 36% between 2002 and 2014 to a total of 50,220 procedures annually, with a further forecasted growth of 42% by 2040 and 101% by 2060 [3,8]. Data from the National Joint Registry in England and Wales reported that on average 4.3% of primary THA will require revision within 10 years [7]. Further analysis showed that of these revisions 10.8% will require a second revision and 1.8% require a third revision [9].

THA are commonly revised for periprosthetic joint infection (PJI), aseptic loosening, instability, peri-prosthetic fracture, and adverse reactions to particulate debris [7,10,11]. Key challenges that need to be overcome in revision THA include establishing stability and restoring hip biomechanics in the presence of bone loss and poor bone quality [10,12]. The rising volume of revision surgery has driven technological advancements in modern implants to both reduce the revision rate of primary THA as well as providing solutions to perform more complex revision THA. First generation designs of uncemented acetabular cups have proven to perform well, with 70.1% to 89.3% survivability at 15 years; however, aseptic loosening remains a common reason for failure [13,14]. With conventional manufacturing methods in uncemented cups, various techniques have been utilised to enhance initial and long-term component stability such as titanium plasma spray, grit blasting, cobalt chrome beads, titanium metal fibre, and hydroxyapatite [15,16].

Over the last decade 'additive manufacturing' has grown in use in manufacturing 3-dimensional (3-D)-printed ultra porous titanium acetabular cups in bulk with a porosity of >60% and mean pore size > 400 nm while maintaining the advantages of titanium [15]. These cups are effectively produced from trabecular titanium [17]. Their characteristics have been proposed to provide increased stability compared to conventional manufacturing methods due to their high porosity, higher coefficient of friction against bone, and a modulus of elasticity nearer to that of bone [12,15,18]. These characteristics of 3-D-printed trabecular titanium components differ to conventionally manufactured components which utilise computer numerical controlled (CNC) machining to create a dense solid dome with various coated surfaces to increase porosity [19].

Additive manufacturing has been proposed as an improvement to conventionally manufactured acetabular implants; however, it is still a relatively new technology with notable differences amongst 3-D-printed titanium acetabular cups currently available. The purpose of this review was to investigate the short- to mid-term clinical and radiographic outcomes of revision THA with ultra porous titanium cups produced with 3-D printing additive manufacturing technology.

2. Materials and Methods

2.1. Search Criteria

The Preferred Reporting Items for Systematic reviews and meta-analyses (PRISMA) criteria was followed to conduct this systematic review [20]. A manual search was performed of the databases of the US National Library of medicine (PubMed/MEDLINE), Embase, and the Cochrane library. The following keywords of "revision total hip arthroplasty" AND "acetabulum" AND "titanium" AND "porous" were utilised. The study protocol was registered in the International Prospective Register of Systematic Reviews (PROSPERO): study number CRD42024565355.

2.2. Inclusion Criteria and Exclusion Criteria

The inclusion criteria were clinical trials investigating revision total hip arthroplasty using off the shelf highly porous titanium acetabular implants manufactured with 3-D printing additive technology. Highly porous was defined as porosity > 60% and >400 microns mean pore size [15].

The exclusion criteria were (1) non-English language studies, (2) studies with less than 10 participants, (3) studies without radiological, clinical or functional outcomes reported, (4) biomechanical studies, (5) reviews or systematic reviews, (6) studies assessing use of cages, cup cages, oblong cups, tantalum metal, or customised implants, (7) studies with less than 2 years mean follow up, (8) non-full-text articles.

2.3. Data Collection

Two authors searched the relevant databases independently and compiled a list of studies matching the inclusion and exclusion criteria. From the studies that were included the following information was tabulated: title, author, year of publication, study design, number of patients/joints, gender, age, BMI, type of acetabular component, classification of acetabular defect, clinical outcomes, radiological outcomes, reason for revision, and complications.

2.4. Assessment of Study Quality

The Methodological Index for Non-Randomized Studies (MINORS) score was used in the assessment of the quality of the studies included. The MINORS score is useful when assessing non-randomized studies, and has been used in many arthroplasty studies. It consists of 8 questions that can be scored individually 0 to 2 [21]. The question is scored as 0 if the relevant information is not included in the study, 1 if it is included but not adequately described and 2 if it is included and described well [21]. The study is graded as poor if the score is lower than 5, moderate with a score of 6–10, and good if the score is 11–16 points. Two authors calculated the scores, with a third author consulted if there was any disagreement (Table 1).

2.5. Statistical Analysis

Continuous variables were presented with range or mean values and standard deviation. Categorical variables were presented with frequency and percentages. Statistical analysis was performed using RStudio Version 4.4.2 (R Foundation for Statistical Computing, Austria). Heterogeneity was assessed using study mean age, sex, follow-up, duration, and implant type using I^2, with $I^2 > 50\%$ considered heterogenous, where random effects methods were preferred. Due to residual heterogeneity (I = 53.46% [95% CI: 8.4–76.3], $p = 0.090$) random effects meta-analysis was used to determine effect size estimates for overall survival and postoperative Harris Hip Score (HHS), weighted by sample size. HHS standard deviation data were approximated from median and range using established techniques in one study [22], and through imputation in one study. The Freeman–Tukey double arcsine transformation was used for all meta-analyses and data were back-transformed prior to interpretation. Effect sizes with 95% confidence intervals were reported for all analyses.

3. Results

3.1. Search Results

Using the keywords described above resulted in the identification of 106 abstracts. (76 in PubMed, 23 in Embase and 7 in Cochrane) (Figure 1). Duplicate articles were identified and removed. The remaining abstracts were screened using the inclusion and exclusion criteria. In total, 18 articles were subjected to further analysis with review of the full text, with a total of 6 articles that fulfilled all criteria and were included in the review. An additional five articles were identified through the citation process that matched the inclusion and exclusion criteria and were therefore included. The level of evidence for all studies was level three with the exception of one case series (Table 1).

Table 1. Type of study, level of evidence and modified Coleman score.

Authors	Type of Study	Quality of Evidence	MINORS Score
Castagnini et al. (2021) [23]	retrospective case series	IV	11
Cozzi Lepri et al. (2022) [10]	retrospective cohort	III	9
De Meo et al. (2018) [11]	retrospective cohort	III	11
Shaarani et al. (2023) [12]	retrospective cohort	III	10
Shang et al. (2022) [24]	retrospective cohort	III	11
Shichman (2022) [25]	retrospective cohort	III	10
El Ghazawy et al. (2022) [26]	retrospective cohort	III	10
Perticarini et al. (2021) [27]	retrospective cohort	III	10
Munegato et al. (2018) [28]	retrospective cohort	III	10
Gallart et al. (2016) [29]	retrospective cohort	III	10
Steno et al. (2015) [17]	retrospective cohort	III	11

3.2. Demographics

In total, 585 patients with 597 operated joints were included in this review. There were 349 (59.7%) female patients. The mean age per study ranged from 56.0 to 78.4 years. The mean body mass index varied between 25.61 and 30.36 kg/m^2. The mean reported follow-up periods ranged between 25.7 months and 91 months (Table 2).

Table 2. Summary of demographic details.

Authors	Number of Hips (Patients)	Gender F	Gender M	Mean Age	Mean BMI (kg/m^2)	Mean Follow Up
Castagnini et al. (2021) [23]	18 (16)	13	3	62.3 ± 8.3 (range 51–83)	26.2 ± 3.1 (range 21.4–31.2)	5.7 years ± 0.7 (range 5–7 years)
Cozzi Lepri et al. (2022) [10]	85	50	35	67.8 (range 32–83)	26.9 (95% confidence interval 25.4–27.7, range 18.3–33)	6.12 years (range 2–10.2)
De Meo et al. (2018) [11]	64	37	27	78.4 (range 42–87)	26.1 (range 23.5–33.2)	48.3 months (range 38–82.3)
Shaarani et al. (2023) [12]	59 (55)	34	25	68.8 SD 12.3	26.6 SD 5.9	25.7 months SD 13.8 (range 4–52)
Shang et al. (2022) [24]	23	13	10	70.35 ± 8.1	25.61 ± 2.80	41.82 months ±11.44 (range 24–64)
Shichman (2022) [25]	40	22	18	71.42 ± 9.97	30.36 ± 6.88	2.21 years ±0.77
El Ghazawy et al. (2022) [26]	24	6	18	56 (range 30–67)	Not stated	20.75 months (14–30)
Perticarini et al. (2021) [27]	95	65	30	70 (range 29–90) SD 11	25.68 (range 17–36.67) SD 3.7	91 months (24–146)
Munegato et al. (2018) [28]	36 (34)	24	14	75 (range 45–92)	Not stated	39.8 months (12–91.5)
Gallart et al. (2016) [29]	72 (69)	34	38	70.7 SD 10.3	Not stated	30.5 months SD 16.9
Steno et al. (2015) [17]	81 (80)	51	30	68.3 (range 32–84)	Not stated	38.14 months (24–62)

SD: Standard deviation.

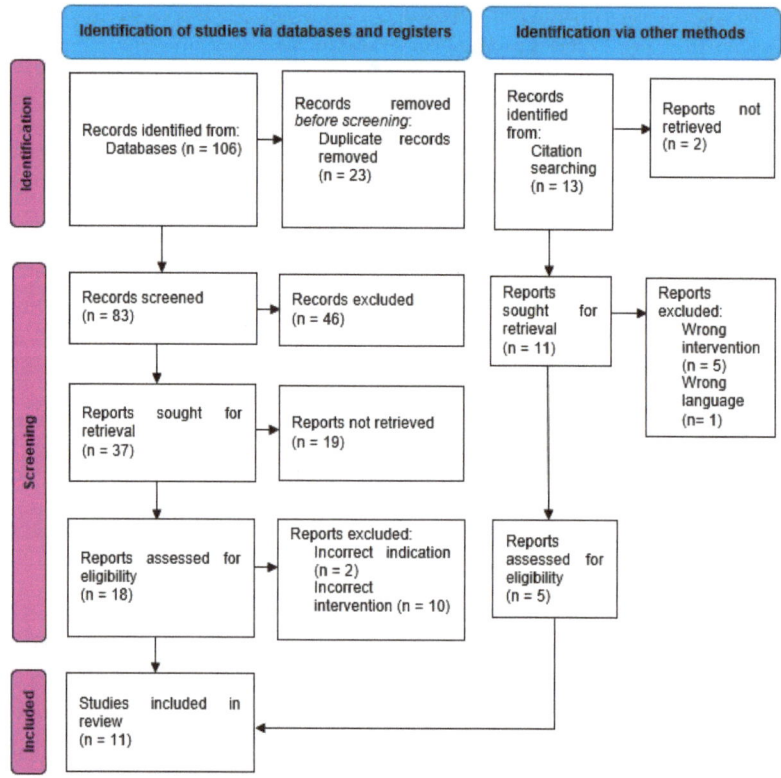

Figure 1. Flow chart of study selection according to PRISMA guidelines [20].

3.3. Indications for Surgery

The most common indications reported for revision surgery were aseptic loosening with 355 cases (59.5%), periprosthetic joint infection (PJI) with 77 cases (12.9%) and instability with 62 cases (10.4%). Other causes included symptomatic elevation of metal ions in metal-on-metal bearing surface, osteolysis, pseudotumour/metalosis, trunnionosis, implant failure and periprosthetic fractures (Table 3).

Table 3. Type of acetabular defects and indications for surgery.

Authors	Acetabular Defects	Indication for Surgery
Castagnini et al. (2021) [23]	Paprosky I 15 (83.3%), Paprosky II 3 (16.7%)	All cases were revisions of Du Puy ASR XL metal on metal bearing surface. 5 (27.8%) aseptic loosening and raised metal ions, 8 (44.4%) pain and metal ions over threshold, 4 (22.2%) osteolysis, 1 (5.6%) pseudotumour.
Cozzi Lepri et al. (2022) [10]	Paprosky IIB 23 (27.1%), Paprosky IIC 20 (23.5%), Paprosky IIIA 24 (28.2%), Paprosky IIIB 18 (21.2%)	31 (36.5%) aseptic loosening, 19 (22.3%) recurrent instability, 15 (17.6%) adverse reaction to metal debris (ARMD), 11 (13%) PJI, 9 (10.6%) periprosthetic fracture.
De Meo et al. (2018) [11]	Paprosky IIB 25 (39%), Paprosky IIC 15 (23.4%), Paprosky IIIA 15 (23.4%), Paprosky IIIB 9 (14.1%)	28 (43.75%) aseptic loosening, 26 (40.6%) instability, 10 (15.6%) wear debris osteolysis.

Table 3. Cont.

Authors	Acetabular Defects	Indication for Surgery
Shaarani et al. (2023) [12]	paprosky I 21 (35.6%), Paprosky IIA 19 (32.2%), Paprosky IIB 3 (5.1%), Paprosky IIC 9 (15.3%), Paprosky IIIA 4 (6.8%), Paprosky IIIB 3 (5.1%)	21 (35.59%) aseptic loosening, 11 (18.64%) PJI, 3 (5.08%) instability, 3 (5.08%) failed DHS, 5 (%) failed hip resurfacing, 2 (3.39%) metastatic disease, 1 (1.69%) acetabular erosion from hemi arthroplasty, 1 (1.69%) squeaking ceramic on ceramic, 1 (1.69%) native hip joint dislocation, 1 (1.69%) broken cement/osteolysis, 1 (1.69%) neck of femur fracture, 1.69%) acetabular fracture, 8 (13.56%) peri-prosthetic fracture, 1 (1.69%) stem fracture.
Shang et al. (2022) [24]	Paprosky I 4 (17.39%), Paprosky II 15 (65.22%), Paprosky III 4 (17.39%)	17 (73.91%) aseptic loosening, 6 (26.09%) PJI.
Shichman (2022) [25]	Paprosky I 1 (2.5%), Paprosky IIA 10 (25%), Paprosky IIB 14 (35.0%), Paprosky IIC 2 (5%), Paprosky IIIB 11 (35%), Paprosky IIIC 2 (5%)	22 (55%) aseptic loosening, 8 (32%) PJI, 2 (5%) instability, 1 (2.5%) trunnionosis, 1 (2.5%) pseudotumour, 6 (15%) complex primary.
El Ghazawy et al. (2022) [26]	Paprosky IIIA 7 (29.2%), Paprosky IIIB 15 (62.5%), Paprosky IIB 2 (8.3%)	19 (79.2%) aseptic loosening, 3 (12.5%) PJI, 2 (8.3%) revision hemiarthroplasty for acetabular erosion.
Perticarini et al. (2021) [27]	Paprosky II 53 (55.8%), Paprosky III 42 (44.2%)	86 (82.69%) aseptic loosening, 8 (7.69%) metallosis, 4 (3.85%) periprosthetic fracture, 3 (2.88%) implant failure, 2 (1.92%) instability, 1 (0.96%) PJI
Munegato et al. (2018) [28]	Paprosky IIB 5 (13.9%), Paprosky IIC 7 (19.4%), Paprosky IIIA 15 (41.7%), Paprosky IIIB 9 (25%)	33 (91.7%) aseptic loosening, 2 (5.6%) PJI, 2 (2.7%) instability.
Gallart et al. (2016) [29]	Paprosky I 19 (26.4%), Paprosky IIA 12 (16.7%), Paprosky IIB 9 (12.5%), Paprosky IIC 16 (22.2%), Paprosky IIIA 12 (16.7%), Paprosky IIIB 4 (5.6%)	31 (43.1%) aseptic loosening, 27 (37.5%) PJI, 4 (5.6%) instability, 3 (4.2%) metallosis, 2 (2.8%) IMN failure, 1 (1.4%) RA, 1 (1.4%) spondyloarthritis.
Steno et al. (2015) [17]	Paprosky type I 9 (11.1%), Paprosky IIA 11 (13.6%), Paprosky IIB 27 (33.3%), Paprosky IIC 6 (7.4%), Paprosky IIIA 15 (18.5%), Paprosky IIIB 13 (16%)	66 (81.5%) aseptic loosening, 3 (3.7%) conversion hemiarthroplasty, 4 (4.9%) instability, 8 (9.9%) PJI.

3.4. Classification of Acetabular Defects

All studies in this review used the Paprosky Classification when describing acetabular defects (Table 3). Paprosky Type I included 69 cases (11.6%), Paprosky Type II 71 cases (11.9%), Paprosky Type IIA 52 cases (8.7%), Paprosky Type IIB 108 cases (18.1%), Paprosky Type IIC 75 cases (12.6%), Paprosky Type III 46 cases (7.7%), Paprosky Type IIIA 92 cases (15.4%), Paprosky Type IIIB 82 cases (13.7%), and Paprosky Type IIIC 2 cases (0.3%).

3.5. Type of Implants

In total, 4 different acetabular systems were reported in the 11 studies (Table 4). In total, 7 studies reported on the use of the Delta (Trabecular Titanium) TT system (Limo Corporate, San Daniele, Italy), including 19 (3.2%) Delta TT, 228 (38.2%) Delta One TT and 210 (35.2%) Delta Revision TT with a total of 457 (76.5%) joints [10,11,17,26–29]. Two studies reported on the REDAPT shell (Smith and Nephew, Memphis, USA) with a total of 99 joints (16.6%) [12,25], one study reported on the Ti-por cup (Adler Ortho, Milan, Italy) with 18 joints (3.0%) [23] and one study reported on the Aikang TT cup (Beijing, China) in 23 joints (3.9%) [24].

A total of 6 studies included information regarding bearing surfaces and head size [10,12,25], with 1 study using dual mobility in all 85 revision cases [10], and 4 other studies employed dual mobility for a proportion of their cohort. Dual mobility was used in a total of 128 cases (21.4%). All studies, with the exception of one, reported on the use of allograft (n = 319, 53.4%), eight studies used augments (n = 84, 14.1%) and two studies used medial wall mesh (n = 16, 2.7%) [10]. Only seven studies reported on the use of screws for cup stabilisation [10,12,23,25].

Table 4. Description of implants, cups, bearings, augments, grafts and screws.

Authors	Manufacturer of Implant	Type of Acetabular Cup	Details of Acetabular Cup Size	Bearing Surfaces	Use of Grafts and Augments	Use of Screws
Castagnini et al. (2021) [23]	Adler	Ti-por cup	50.6 mm ± 3.6 (range 46–56) (Mean)	not specified	3 (16.7%) morselise bone allograft	3 cases (16.7%)
Cozzi Lepri et al. (2022) [10]	Lima	Delta TT one in 30 (35.3%), Delta TT revision in 55 (64.7%)	not specified	85 (100%) Dual mobility	85 (100%), corticocancellous allograft, 12 (14.11%) medial wall meshes	4.2 (range 2–7) (Mean)
De Meo et al. (2018) [11]	Lima	Delta TT one in 39 (60.9%), Delta TT revision in 25 (39.1%)	not specified	not specified	34 (53.1%), morselise bone allograft, 4 (6.3%) augment	not specified
Shaarani et al. (2023) [12]	Smith and Nephew	REDAPT shell	54 mm (Mode)	29 (49.15%) Dual mobility	6 (10.17%) augment	4 (Median)
Shang et al. (2022) [24]	Aikang corp	Aikang TT	not specified	not specified	4 (17.39%) augment, 1 (4.35%) structural bone graft, 5 (21.74%) augment and bone graft	not specified
Shichman (2022) [25]	Smith and Nephew	REDAPT shell	60 mm (range 48–80) (Median)	36 mm (range 28–36) (Median)	12 (30%) Allograft	4 (range 2–8) (Median)
El Ghazawy et al. (2022) [26]	Lima	Delta TT revision	Not stated	Head size not stated, 3 (12.5%) Dual mobility	20 (83%) Morselised allograft, 19 (80%) augments	3 (range 2–4) (mean)
Perticarini et al. (2021) [27]	Lima	Delta revision TT in 39 (41.1%), Delta One TT in 56 (58.9%)	46–66 mm	6 (6.3%) Dual mobility	57 (60%) Allograft, 13 (13.7%) augments, 4 (4.2%) meshes	2–6 screws (range)
Munegato et al. (2018) [28]	Lima	Delta TT revision	Not stated	Not stated	24 (66.7%) Allograft, 11 (30.6%) synthetic bone graft	not stated
Gallart et al. (2016) [29]	Lima	Delta Revision TT 18 (25%), Delta One TT 54 (75%)	Not stated	Not stated	22 (30.6%) Allograft, 17 (23.6%) augment	not stated
Steno et al. (2015) [17]	Lima	Delta TT 19 (23.5%), Delta One TT 49 (60.5%), Delta Revision TT 13 (16%)	Mode 58 (range 44–68)	5 (6.2%) Dual mobility	53 (65.4%) Morselised allograft, 3 (3.7%) structural allograft, 16 (19.8%) augments	2–5 screws (range)

3.6. Clinical Outcomes

All patient reported outcome measures improved postoperatively in all studies (Table 5). The most common reported clinical outcome measure reported was the HHS, which was used in eight studies (n = 385, 64.5%) [10,11,23–28]. Meta-analysis of HHS was calculated as a mean of 86.7 (95% CI: 84.3–89.1). One study used the Short-form 36 (SF-36) (mean 754.04, standard deviation [SD] 22.74) and the Visual Analogue Scale

(VAS) (1.14 SD 0.23) in combination with HHS [24], and another study used length of stay (LOS) (5.34 days ± 3.34) [25]. One study used the Oxford hip score (OHS) (83, SD 15) and Short-form 12 (SF-12) physical (44, SD 11), SF-12 mental (56 SD 10), Western Ontario and McMaster Universities Osteoarthritis Index (WOMAC) (85 SD 17) [12]. Two studies used Merle d'Aubigné-Postel scores [17,29].

3.7. Imaging Outcomes

All studies reported on radiological outcomes. One study used the criteria according to Moore et al. (2006) to assess osteointegration [23,30]. Two studies used Gie et al. (1993) to report on bone graft incorporation [10,28,31]. Four studies reported no radiolucencies on post-operative radiographs at follow-up, and two studies reported six (1.0%) cup migrations (Table 5).

3.8. Survival and Complication Rates

Meta-analysis of all-cause cup survival was 95.52% (95% CI: 92.37–97.96) at a mean follow up of 3.8 years (95% CI: 2.6–5.1). In total, 80 (13.4%) complications were reported with 40 (6.7%) complications not requiring re-operation that included deep vein thrombosis (DVT) (n = 20, 3.4%), wound problems (n = 3, 0.5%), instability (n = 3, 0.5%), cup migration (n = 4, 0.7%), heterotrophic ossification (n = 3, 0.5%), femoral neurapraxia (n = 4, 0.7%), psoas tendinopathy (n = 1, 0.2%), persistent pain (n = 1, 0.2%), and trochanteric bursitis (n = 1, 0.2%). In total, 40 cases (6.7%) required re-operation with causes including 17 (2.8%) cases of PJI, 14 (2.3%) cases of instability, 5 (0.8%) cases of aseptic loosening and 2 (0.3%) cases of shell migration (Table 5).

Table 5. Clinical and radiological outcome measures, survival rate and complications.

Authors	Clinical Outcomes	Radiological Outcomes	Survival Rate	Complications	Causes for Re-Operation
Castagnini et al. (2021) [23]	HHS 88.3 ± 9.2 (range 68–97)	No cup loosening or cup migration at final follow up. No periacetabular radiolucency. Good cup osseointegration according to Moore et al. (2006) [30] of >3 in every case.	100%	4 complications in 3 (16.7%) cases. 1 (5.6%) PJI, 1 (5.6%) wound infection, 1 (5.6%) dislocation, 1 (5.6%) psoas tendonitis	No revision
Cozzi Lepri et al. (2022) [10]	HHS 89.7 (range 83–98)	Bone graft incorporation according to Gie et al. (1993) [31] type 1 (n = 8, 9.4%), type 2 (n = 22, 25.9%), type 3 (n = 55, 64.7%).	5 year 100%, 10 year 88%	19 (22.4%) DVT, 4 (4.7%) femoral neuropraxia, 1 (1.2%) aseptic loosening, 1 (1.2%) PJI	2 (2.3%) cases re-operation after 5.6 years. 1 (1.2%) aseptic loosening
De Meo et al. (2018) [11]	HHS 83.7 (range 58.9–91.3)	No radiolucent lines or signs of migration were observed.	Kaplan–Meier survivorship curve at 48.3 months showed survivorship of 89.7% for revision and 94.8% for acetabular cup removal	3 (5.2%) instability, 2 (3.4%) PJI, 1 (1.7%) aseptic loosening	6 (10.3%) cases re-operation. 3 (5.2%) instability, 2 (3.4%) PJI (3.4%), 1 (1.7%) aseptic loosening
Shaarani et al. (2023) [12]	OHS 83 (SD 15), SF-12 physical 44 (SD 11), SF-12 mental 56 (SD 10), WOMAC function score 84 (SD 17), WOMAC stiffness score 83 (SD 15), WOMAC pain score 85 (SD 15), WOMAC global score 85 (SD 17)	2 (3.4%) Shell migration, no radiographs demonstrated radiolucency.	-	2 (3.4%) shell migrations, 1 (1.7%) acute PJI	1 (1.7%) revision of liner for PJI. 1 (1.7%) planned revision of cup migration
Shang et al. (2022) [24]	HHS 90.48 SD 3.65, SF-36 754.04 SD 22.74, VAS 1.14 SD 0.23	All cups remained stable with no loosening and no changes in cup abduction angle. According to bone growth criteria from Anderson Orthopaedic Research institute, 2 cups had 2 signs, 17 had 3 signs, 4 had 4 signs.	100%	1 (4.3%) persistent pain, 1 (4.3%) persistent wound drainage	No revisions
Shichman (2022) [25]	HHS 83.53 ± 12.15, LOS 5.34 ± 3.34,	39/40 (97.5%) cups had osteointegration, 1 (2.5%) reported cup migration.	Kaplan-Meier showed all-cause revision free survival rate of 95.0% at 6 months and 1 year, and 92.0% at 4 years	2 (5%) Acute PJI, 1 (2.5%) implant migration with aseptic loosening, 1 (2.5%) DVT	1 (2.5%) Implant migration with aseptic loosening, 2 (5%) PJI

Table 5. *Cont.*

Authors	Clinical Outcomes	Radiological Outcomes	Survival Rate	Complications	Causes for Re-Operation
El Ghazawy et al. (2022) [26]	HHS 85 (range 70–98)	No change in cup position. No progressive radiolucency.	100%	No complications	No re-operations
Perticarini et al. (2021) [27]	HHS 84.4 (range 46–99) SD 7.56	1 (1.1%) graft resorption. All other cups no cup migration or aseptic loosening.	88.54% (95 CI 80.18–93.52%) at 71 months	7 (7.3%) PJI, 7 (7.3%) Instability, 1(1.1%) graft resorption with aseptic loosening, 2 (2.1%) periprosthetic femur fracture, 1 (1.1%) trochanteric bursitis, 3 (3.2%) heterotrophic ossification	7 (7.3%) PJI, 5 (5.3%) instability, 1 (1.1%) graft resorption with aseptic loosening, 2 (2.1%) periprosthetic femur fracture
Munegato et al. (2018) [28]	HHS 87 (SD ± 7.7)	No signs of loosening, bone graft graded to Gie: 21 (58.3%) Type 3, 12 (33.3%) Type 2, 2 (5.6%) Type 1.	100% for aseptic loosening, 91.7% for any revision	1 (2.8%) PJI, 2 (5.6%) instability	1 (2.8%) PJI with dislocation, 2 (5.6%) cases of instability that developed PJI after re-operation
Gallart et al. (2016) [29]	Merle d'Aubigné-Postel score pain 5.7 ± 0.7, walking 5.3 ± 0.7, range of motion 5.6 ± 0.7	Not stated.	88.89%	3 (4.2%) PJI, 3 (4.2%) Instability, 2 (2.8) aseptic loosening	3 (4.2%) PJI, 3 (4.2%) Instability, 2 (2.8) aseptic loosening
Steno et al. (2015) [17]	Merle d'Aubigné-Postel functional score 9.78, pain 5.45 (range 3–6), walking 4.33 (range 3–6)	3 (3.7%) initial cup migrations that stabilised with no radiolucency at final follow up.	98.77%	3 (3.7%) cups with medial migration that stabilised, 1 (1.2%) instability	1 (1.2%) instability

4. Discussion

When compared to primary THA, revision THA is associated with an increased risk of complications and places increased physiological, psychological and economic burdens on both the patient, healthcare providers and the healthcare system [24,32]. Revision surgery is complex and is fraught with technical difficulties in dealing with poor bone quality and bone defects. Acetabular components are more frequently revised than stems in isolated component revisions [33]. The overall success rates for revision THA ranges from 61.3% to 98.3% [34]. Uncemented implants have shown better success rates compared to cemented components in revision THA [17]. Finding the balance between stable acetabular cup fixation and restoration of the hip biomechanical parameters is necessary for improved success in revision THA [10]. Porous metals have been the most recent advance in surface technology, with creation of 3-D structures of interconnected porous channels similar to trabecular bone to achieve this balance [16]. Initially, tantalum was used in the manufacturing of these highly porous components of trabecular metal with well-established favourable short- and mid-term survival [16,27,35]. However, tantalum is a rare metal with far less available for 3-D printing applications compared to titanium due to technical and economic factors [36]. Additive manufacturing using 3-D printing techniques, with a –aluminium–vanadium (Ti-6Al-4 V) alloy powder, has evolved from traditional manufacturing methods of "formative shaping" or "subtractive manufacturing" using titanium with various techniques of coating [24].

Additive manufacturing results in up to 75% reduction in raw material usage and up to 50% reduction in the costs of the manufacturing process [37]. Additive manufacturing combines the beneficial properties of titanium, including biocompatibility, strength and resistance to corrosion, with the benefits of high porosity components in bulk production of readily available implants [13,14,32]. Three-dimensional printing techniques may use Electron Beam Melting (EBM) or Selective Laser Melting (SLM) to produce highly porous components with specific pore size, shape and density [11,24]. This effectively results in titanium trabecular metal implants, which have technical parameters that are similar to those of more established tantalum implants with mean pore size of 550 μm and porosity of 75–80% [10,35]. Highly porous titanium acetabular shells have elasticity and a microstructure similar to bone, improving the initial and long-term stability with a high coefficient of friction and a structure promoting osseointegration [13,25].

There are a growing number of manufacturers using additive manufacturing technology in creating acetabular components (Table 6). The use of 'off the shelf' highly porous 3-D-printed titanium acetabular shells for revision arthroplasty surgery has been evaluated in only a few studies. This current review provides evidence that highly porous 3-D-printed titanium acetabular shells resulted in good early to mid-term outcomes when employed for revision THA, with an all-cause survivorship of 95.52%, with four studies reporting 100% survivorship at mean follow-up of 1.7 years, 3.5 years, 5 years and 5.7 years.

Table 6. Comparison of components using additive manufacturing.

Manufacturer	Acetabular Cup	Composition	Tradename Porous Structure	Porosity (%)	Pore Diameter (μm)	Production Method	References:
Lima Corporate (San Daniele, Italy)	Delta TT cup	Titanium	Trabecular titanium	65	640	EBM	[37,38]
	Delta revision TT	Titanium	Trabecular titanium	65	640	EBM	[37,38]
	Delta one TT	Titanium	Trabecular titanium	65	640	EBM	[37,38]
Smith and Nephew (Memphis, TN, USA)	REDAPT	Titanium	Conceloc Advanced Porous Titanium	60–80	200–934	EBM	[14,37]
Aikang Corp. (Beijing, China)	3D ACT	Titanium	-	80	600–1000	EBM	[24]
Adler Ortho (Milan, Italy)	Omnia	Titanium	Tri-Por Cup	65–70	700	EBM	[14,37]
	Polymax ti-por	Titanium	Tri-Por Cup	65–70	700	EBM	[14,37]
	Omnia ti-por	Titanium	Tri-Por Cup	65–70	700	EBM	[14,37]
	Fixa ti-por	Titanium	Tri-Por Cup	65–70	700	EBM	[14,37]
	Agilis ti-por	Titanium	Tri-Por Cup	65–70	700	EBM	[14,37]
Stryker (Mahwah, NJ, USA)	Trident II	Titanium	Tritanium	55–65	100–700	SLM	[14,37,38]
Zimmer (Warsaw, IN, USA)	G7	Titanium	OsseoTi porous technology	70	475	-	[14,37]
Medacta (Castel San Pietro, Switzerland)	Mpact 3D metal	Titanium	3D Metal	75	600–800	EBM	[37,38]
Kyocera (Kyoto, Japan)	SQRUM TT	Titanium	-	60	640	EBM	[18,37]
Implantcast (Buxtehude, Germany)	Ecofit Epore	Titanium	EPORE	60	100–500	EBM	[14,37]
Corin (Cirencester, UK)	Trinity Plus	Titanium	PLUS (Porous layer unique structure)	50–90	300–900	-	[37]

It is difficult to make direct comparisons between studies reporting the outcomes of revision THA due to the heterogenicity of indications, varying morphology of bone defects and the combinations of implant usage available [25]. Vutescu et al. (2017) made adjustments for acetabular defect severity when comparing more established trabecular tantalum to ultra porous titanium implants used in revision THA, and found no difference, with both implants resulting in excellent outcomes at 5 years [16]. Previous systematic reviews have assessed the outcomes of 3-D-printed titanium cups; however, to the authors knowledge, this is the first review assessing the use of different types of 3-D-printed titanium implants for revision THA. The majority of the implants reported in this review used the Delta TT system (Lima corporate, San Daniele, Italy). This system has been available since 2007, giving it the longest period of availability for use [29].

Cacciola et al. (2023) previously reviewed 3-D-printed titanium acetabular implants and reported an overall survival rate of 93.4%, similar to the findings of this study of 95.52% [39]. They included a total of 523 hip revisions from eight studies; however, they only included Delta TT systems (Lima corporate) in their review [39]. Instability was the most common complication of 4.1%, with aseptic loosening of 1.5%, which differs from the results of the current review, with PJI being the most common complication followed by instability requiring re-operation. The majority of the studies from Cacciola et al. (2023) were included in the current systematic review, which also included the results from the Delta Revision TT cup [39]. This revision cup is 3-D printed using EBM but differs from Delta One TT and Delta TT cups, and all other hemispherical titanium cups, due to a "cage construct" with a built-in hook and three 'winglets' [17]. Whether these have a significant clinical impact on implant survival is still to be determined, although most studies report their use in more severe defects which may bias outcomes. Gallart et al. reported no difference ($p = 0.101$) in failures of aseptic loosening with Delta One cups compared to Delta TT Revision components [29]. Future studies comparing these cups to standard hemispherical designs as well as other trabecular metal designs are needed.

The systematic review by Malahias et al. (2019) assessed highly porous titanium acetabular cups in both primary and revision settings. It was reported that in revision THA, there was an overall acetabular revision rate of 6.5% [15]. The rates of aseptic loosening of the acetabular component (2.4%), PJI (2.4%) and dislocations (2.4%) were also found to be low and comparable to the findings of this current review [15]. There was improvement in all clinical scores [15]. Although the inclusion criteria were specific with mean porosity and mean pore size similar to components manufactured with 3-D printing, the study also included ultra-high porosity implants that were not 3-D printed with additive technology such as the Trident acetabular cup (Stryker), the predecessor to the Trident II acetabular cup (Stryker, Mahwah, USA) [15]. These are highly porous titanium acetabular cups used in revision THA and have shown survivorship ranging from 91% to 98.4% after at least 5 years [40–42]. Although the cups reported had similar surface characteristics of mean pore size and pore density, they are manufactured with conventional techniques and lack the proposed advantages of 3-D-printed trabecular titanium [15].

Tsikandylakis et al. (2020) reported their randomised control trial comparing 3-D-printed titanium cups to cups conventionally manufactured with porous plasma spray (PPS) [33]. It was found that 3-D-printed cups were not superior in cup fixation within the 2-year follow-up period in respect to radiological and clinical outcomes, but only primary THA cases were assessed [33]. In this current review, only one study compared 3-D-printed cups to non-3-D-printed cups used in revision THA, which demonstrated that 3-D-printed cups had better HHS and SF-36 scores and had significantly better bone ingrowth than conventionally manufactured cups [24]. The difference in findings between these two studies may be due to the difference of comparing primary versus revision THA, and that the benefits of 3-D-printed cups are more pronounced in settings of compromised bone quality and quantity. This is similar to the difference found between trabecular metal tantalum cups and hydroxyapatite-coated titanium cups by Meneghini et al., with a more pronounced difference in outcomes noted in major bone deficiency compared to minor defects [17,43]. The systematic review with meta-analysis by Shen et al. (2022) found a survival rate of 92.5% at 10-year follow up for tantalum cups, and when comparing tantalum to titanium implants, it was found tantalum acetabular cups had fewer complications of aseptic loosening and PJI, but more dislocations compared to titanium cups [44]. These cups were not 3-D printed [44]. There are obviously differences noted between all these implants. More studies directly comparing 3-D printed titanium implants to conventionally manufactured titanium implants to, as well as to tantalum implants used in revision THA are needed.

Only six studies reported on the type of bearing surface and five studies reported on cup size; however, the parameters used were inconsistent, making comparisons difficult. One reported advantage of 3-D-printed titanium acetabular cups is the cup size optimisation due to the thinner implant thickness of these components [14]. Information regarding the cup size, polyethylene liner size and head size as well as the bearing surface used may be beneficial to include in future studies to determine the clinical significance of these parameters.

All studies in this review reported on the use of augments and bone grafts, but only seven studies reported on the use of screws. Shaarani et al. (2023) found that there was an increase in the quantity of screws with increased age [12]. This relationship may suggest that there were increased screws in the presence of decreased bone quality; however, since bone quality is difficult to objectively quantify this proposed relationship cannot be confirmed. The details of the types of graft used were not always included, although Strahl et al. (2023) found no significant difference in success rates between the use of different allografts, including bulk structural grafts and morselised grafts in a recent systematic review [34]. These findings need to be interpreted with caution as the type of bone graft used is largely dictated by the morphology of the bone defect present.

Shaarani et al. (2023) reported a negative correlation between cup size and augments [12]. This suggests that large cups, including 'jumbo cups' were used to adequately address bone defects without the use of augments; however, this was found to be at the expense of raising the hip centre of rotation [12]. Unfortunately, none of the studies examined the impact of bone graft, augments, screws, cup size and bearing surfaces on clinical outcomes and incidence of complications. The difficulty of this is not underestimated, as the usage of bone grafts, augments and screws usually indirectly indicates the complexity of the case with the quantity and quality of bone available. Further studies evaluating the combinations of these components used with 3-D-printed titanium cups in revision THA setting are needed.

Contact between host bone and the implant surface is crucial for the success of acetabular components in revision THA [29]. The necessary surface area contact may differ between implants depending on the qualities of the implant including biocompatibility, strength, elasticity, and mean pore size and porosity [10,32]. Bone loss was classified according to Paprosky by all studies in this review, with Paprosky type IIB being the most common pattern of bone loss reported, followed by Type IIIA, Type IIIB and Type IIC. Outcomes and failures were not matched according to bone loss defects in the majority of studies.

Gallart et al. compared acetabular component failures according to the Paprosky classification. Paprosky type 1 had no failures, and more severe bone defects of Paproksy type II and type III had four failures each ($p = 0.028$) [29]. When interpreting these results, it should be noted that allograft or augments were used in the majority of Paprosky Type II defects whilst Delta Revision TT cups with built in flanges were used in Paprosky type III [29].

Steno et al. (2015) reported no acetabular cup migrations except for three cases in which Delta Revision TT was combined with allograft in Paprosky type IIIB defects, with all other defects having 100% survival and no cup migrations [17]. Comparing outcomes to the bone defects and the type of implants used in future larger studies may be beneficial in providing insights into the limit of usage of different implants.

The limitations of this review relate to the quality of the studies being examined. There are no level 1 or level 2 data available, and the use of inclusion/exclusion criteria is variable. The difference in study designs, patient populations and follow-up periods makes comparative research difficult. There were no prospective studies available and average values, SD and ranges were reported inconsistently by the various included studies. The use of different outcome measures in both clinical assessment and radiological assessment made comparative research challenging.

5. Conclusions

Revision THA are complex procedures often with diminished bone quality and quantity available for component fixation. The evolution of a new generation of titanium acetabular implants using 3-D printing additive manufacturing techniques have resulted in excellent short- to mid-term outcomes in this review. Future prospective long-term studies, with standardization of both clinical and radiological assessment tools, are needed to compare the success and longevity of these implants to other more established options such as tantalum trabecular metal and readily available conventionally manufactured titanium implants.

Author Contributions: Conceptualization, N.D.C. and P.R.A.; methodology, N.D.C. and P.R.A.; formal analysis, N.D.C. and P.R.A.; investigation, N.D.C. and P.R.A.; writing—original draft preparation, P.R.A.; writing—review and editing, P.R.A., G.J.M., P.S., P.G. and N.D.C.; All authors have read and agreed to the published version of the manuscript.

Funding: This research received no external funding.

Institutional Review Board Statement: Not applicable.

Informed Consent Statement: Not applicable due to the nature of the study.

Data Availability Statement: All data are available within the text of this systematic review.

Conflicts of Interest: The authors declare no conflicts of interest.

Abbreviations

The following abbreviations are used in this manuscript:

THA	Total hip arthroplasty
3-D	3-dimensional
CNC	computer numerical controlled
PRISMA	Preferred Reporting Items for Systematic reviews and meta-analyses
MINORS	Methodological Index for Non-Randomized Studies
HHS	Harris Hip Score
VAS	Visual Analogue scale
OHS	Oxford hip score
LOS	Length of stay
SF-12	Short-form 12
WOMAC	Western Ontario and McMaster Universities Osteoarthritis Index
EBM	Electron Beam Melting
SLM	Selective Laser Melting

References

1. Blom, A.W.; Donovan, R.L.; Beswick, A.D.; Whitehouse, M.R.; Kunutsor, S.K. Common elective orthopaedic procedures and their clinical effectiveness: Umbrella review of level 1 evidence. *BMJ* **2021**, *374*, n1511. [CrossRef] [PubMed]
2. Learmonth, I.D.; Young, C.; Rorabeck, C. The operation of the century: Total hip replacement. *Lancet* **2007**, *370*, 1508–1519. [CrossRef] [PubMed]
3. Schwartz, A.M.; Farley, K.X.; Guild, G.N.; Bradbury, T.L. Projections and Epidemiology of Revision Hip and Knee Arthroplasty in the United States to 2030. *J. Arthroplast.* **2020**, *35*, S79–S85. [CrossRef]
4. Singh, J.A.; Yu, S.; Chen, L.; Cleveland, J.D. Rates of Total Joint Replacement in the United States: Future Projections to 2020–2040 Using the National Inpatient Sample. *J. Rheumatol.* **2019**, *46*, 1134–1140. [CrossRef] [PubMed]
5. Kurtz, S.; Ong, K.; Lau, E.; Mowat, F.; Halpern, M. Projections of primary and revision hip and knee arthroplasty in the United States from 2005 to 2030. *J. Bone Joint Surg. Am.* **2007**, *89*, 780–785. [CrossRef]
6. Shichman, I.; Roof, M.; Askew, N.; Nherera, L.; Rozell, J.C.; Seyler, T.M.; Schwarzkopf, R. Projections and Epidemiology of Primary Hip and Knee Arthroplasty in Medicare Patients to 2040–2060. *JBJS Open Access* **2023**, *8*, e22. [CrossRef]
7. Deere, K.; Whitehouse, M.R.; Kunutsor, S.K.; Sayers, A.; Mason, J.; Blom, A.W. How long do revised and multiply revised hip replacements last? A retrospective observational study of the National Joint Registry. *Lancet Rheumatol.* **2022**, *4*, e468–e479. [CrossRef] [PubMed]
8. Shichman, I.; Askew, N.; Habibi, A.; Nherera, L.; Macaulay, W.; Seyler, T.; Schwarzkopf, R. Projections and Epidemiology of Revision Hip and Knee Arthroplasty in the United States to 2040-2060. *Arthroplast. Today* **2023**, *21*, 101152. [CrossRef]
9. Karachalios, T.; Komnos, G.; Koutalos, A. Total hip arthroplasty: Survival and modes of failure. *EFORT Open Rev.* **2018**, *3*, 232–239. [CrossRef] [PubMed]
10. Cozzi Lepri, A.; Innocenti, M.; Galeotti, A.; Carulli, C.; Villano, M.; Civinini, R. Trabecular titanium cups in acetabular revision arthroplasty: Analysis of 10-year survivorship, restoration of center of rotation and osteointegration. *Arch. Orthop. Trauma. Surg.* **2022**, *142*, 3523–3531. [CrossRef] [PubMed]
11. De Meo, F.; Cacciola, G.; Bellotti, V.; Bruschetta, A.; Cavaliere, P. Trabecular Titanium acetabular cups in hip revision surgery: Mid-term clinical and radiological outcomes. *HIP Int.* **2018**, *28* (Suppl. S2), 61–65. [CrossRef]
12. Shaarani, S.R.; Jaibaji, M.; Yaghmour, K.M.; Vles, G.; Haddad, F.S.; Konan, S. Early clinical and radiological outcomes of the new porous titanium shell in combination with locking screw in revision total hip arthroplasty. *Arthroplasty* **2023**, *5*, 24. [CrossRef] [PubMed]
13. Castagnini, F.; Bordini, B.; Stea, S.; Calderoni, P.P.; Masetti, C.; Busanelli, L. Highly porous titanium cup in cementless total hip arthroplasty: Registry results at eight years. *Int. Orthop.* **2019**, *43*, 1815–1821. [CrossRef] [PubMed]
14. Dall'Ava, L.; Hothi, H.; Di Laura, A.; Henckel, J.; Hart, A. 3D printed acetabular cups for total hip arthroplasty: A review article. *Metals* **2019**, *9*, 729. [CrossRef]
15. Malahias, M.A.; Kostretzis, L.; Greenberg, A.; Nikolaou, V.S.; Atrey, A.; Sculco, P.K. Highly Porous Titanium Acetabular Components in Primary and Revision Total Hip Arthroplasty: A Systematic Review. *J. Arthroplast.* **2020**, *35*, 1737–1749. [CrossRef] [PubMed]
16. Vutescu, E.S.; Hsiue, P.; Paprosky, W.; Nandi, S. Comparative survival analysis of porous tantalum and porous titanium acetabular components in total hip arthroplasty. *HIP Int.* **2017**, *27*, 505–508. [CrossRef] [PubMed]
17. Steno, B.; Kokavec, M.; Necas, L. Acetabular revision arthroplasty using trabecular titanium implants. *Int. Orthop.* **2015**, *39*, 389–395. [CrossRef]
18. Kaneko, T.; Nakamura, S.; Hayakawa, K.; Tokimura, F.; Miyazaki, T. Clinical and radiological outcomes of total hip arthroplasty in octogenarian patients using a three-dimensional porous titanium cup: A retrospective analysis in Japanese patients. *Eur. J. Orthop. Surg. Traumatol.* **2023**, *33*, 2361–2367. [CrossRef] [PubMed]
19. Dall'ava, L.; Hothi, H.; Henckel, J.; Di Laura, A.; Tirabosco, R.; Eskelinen, A.; Skinner, J.; Hart, A. Osseointegration of retrieved 3D-printed, off-the-shelf acetabular implants Aims. *Bone Joint Res.* **2021**, *10*, 388–400. [CrossRef] [PubMed]
20. Page, M.J.; McKenzie, J.E.; Bossuyt, P.M.; Boutron, I.; Hoffmann, T.C.; Mulrow, C.D.; Shamseer, L.; Tetzlaff, J.M.; Akl, E.A.; Brennan, S.E.; et al. The PRISMA 2020 statement: An updated guideline for reporting systematic reviews. *BMJ* **2021**, *372*, n71. [CrossRef] [PubMed]
21. Slim, K.; Nini, E.; Forestier, D.; Kwiatkowski, F.; Panis, Y.; Chipponi, J. Methodological index for non-randomized studies (Minors): Development and validation of a new instrument. *ANZ J. Surg.* **2003**, *73*, 712–716. [CrossRef] [PubMed]
22. Wan, X.; Wang, W.; Liu, J.; Tong, T. Estimating the sample mean and standard deviation from the sample size, median, range and/or interquartile range. *BMC Med. Res. Methodol.* **2014**, *14*, 135. [CrossRef]
23. Castagnini, F.; Mariotti, F.; Tassinari, E.; Bordini, B.; Zuccheri, F.; Traina, F. lsolated acetabular revisions of articular surface replacement (ASR) XL implants with highly porous titanium cups and Delta bearings. *HIP Int.* **2021**, *31*, 250–257. [CrossRef] [PubMed]

24. Shang, G.; Xiang, S.; Guo, C.; Guo, J.; Wang, P.; Wang, Y.; Xu, H. Use of a new off-the-shelf 3D-printed trabecular titanium acetabular cup in Chinese patients undergoing hip revision surgery: Short- to mid-term clinical and radiological outcomes. *BMC Musculoskelet Disord.* **2022**, *23*, 636. [CrossRef] [PubMed]
25. Shichman, I.; Somerville, L.; Lutes, W.B.; Jones, S.A.; McCalden, R.; Schwarzkopf, R. Outcomes of novel 3D-printed fully porous titanium cup and a cemented highly cross-linked polyethylene liner in complex and revision total hip arthroplasty. *Arthroplasty* **2022**, *4*, 51. [CrossRef] [PubMed]
26. El Ghazawy, A.K.; Bassiony, A.A.; Abdelazim, H.; Gameel, S. Acetabular revision using trabecular titanium (Delta TT) revision cups: A retrospective case series. *SICOT J.* **2022**, *8*, 49. [CrossRef] [PubMed]
27. Perticarini, L.; Rossi, S.M.P.; Medetti, M.; Benazzo, F. Clinical and radiological outcomes of acetabular revision surgery with trabecular titanium cups in Paprosky type II and III bone defects. *J. Orthop. Traumatol.* **2021**, *22*, 9. [CrossRef]
28. Munegato, D.; Bigoni, M.; Sotiri, R.; Bruschetta, A.; Omeljaniuk, R.J.; Turati, M.; Andrea, R.; Zatti, G. Clinical and radiological outcomes of acetabular revision with the Delta Revision TT cup. *HIP Int.* **2018**, *28* (Suppl. S2), 54–60. [CrossRef] [PubMed]
29. Gallart, X.; Fernández-Valencia, J.A.; Riba, J.; Bori, G.; García, S.; Tornero, E.; Combalía, A. Trabecular Titanium™ cups and augments in revision total hip arthroplasty: Clinical results, radiology and survival outcomes. *HIP Int.* **2016**, *26*, 486–491. [CrossRef] [PubMed]
30. Moore, M.S.; McAuley, J.P.; Young, A.M.; Engh, C.A. Radiographic signs of osseointegration in porous-coated acetabular components. *Clin. Orthop. Relat. Res.* **2006**, *444*, 176–183. [CrossRef]
31. Gie, G.A.; Linder, L.; Ling, R.S.M.; Simon, J.P.; Slooff, T.J.J.H.; Timperley, A.J. Impacted Cancellous Allografts And Cement For Revision Total Hip Arthroplasty. *J. Bone Jt. Surg. Br. Vol.* **1993**, *75*, 14–21. [CrossRef] [PubMed]
32. Apostu, D.; Lucaciu, O.; Berce, C.; Lucaciu, D.; Cosma, D. Current methods of preventing aseptic loosening and improving osseointegration of titanium implants in cementless total hip arthroplasty: A review. *J. Int. Med. Res.* **2018**, *46*, 2104–2119. [CrossRef] [PubMed]
33. Tsikandylakis, G.; Mortensen, K.R.L.; Gromov, K.; Troelsen, A.; Malchau, H.; Mohaddes, M. The Use of Porous Titanium Coating and the Largest Possible Head Do Not Affect Early Cup Fixation. *JBJS Open Access* **2020**, *5*, E2000107. [CrossRef] [PubMed]
34. Strahl, A.; Boese, C.K.; Ries, C.; Hubert, J.; Beil, F.T.; Rolvien, T. Outcome of different reconstruction options using allografts in revision total hip arthroplasty for severe acetabular bone loss: A systematic review and meta-analysis. *Arch. Orthop. Trauma. Surg.* **2023**, *143*, 6403–6422. [CrossRef]
35. Argyropoulou, E.; Sakellariou, E.; Galanis, A.; Karampinas, P.; Rozis, M.; Koutas, K.; Tsalimas, G.; Vasiliadis, E.; Vlamis, J.; Pneumaticos, S. Porous Tantalum Acetabular Cups in Primary and Revision Total Hip Arthroplasty: What Has Been the Experience So Far?—A Systematic Literature Review. *Biomedicines* **2024**, *12*, 959. [CrossRef]
36. Ma, K.; Ma, Z.; Cheng, L.; Zhao, D. Progress in the Application of Porous Tantalum Metal in Hip Joint Surgery. *Orthop. Surg.* **2024**, *16*, 2877–2886. [CrossRef] [PubMed]
37. Castagnini, F.; Caternicchia, F.; Biondi, F.; Masetti, C.; Faldini, C.; Traina, F. Off-the-shelf 3D printed titanium cups in primary total hip arthroplasty. *World J. Orthop.* **2021**, *12*, 376–385. [CrossRef]
38. Dall'Ava, L.; Hothi, H.; Henckel, J.; Di Laura, A.; Shearing, P.; Hart, A. Comparative analysis of current 3D printed acetabular titanium implants. *3D Print Med.* **2019**, *5*, 15. [CrossRef] [PubMed]
39. Cacciola, G.; Giustra, F.; Bosco, F.; De Meo, F.; Bruschetta, A.; De Martino, I.; Risitano, S.; Sabatini, L.; Massè, A.; Cavaliere, P. Trabecular titanium cups in hip revision surgery: A systematic review of the literature. *Ann. Jt.* **2023**, *8*, 36. [CrossRef] [PubMed]
40. Ramappa, M.; Bajwa, A.; Kulkarni, A.; Mcmurtry, I.; Port, A. Early results of a new highly porous modular acetabular cup in revision arthroplasty. *Hip Int.* **2009**, *19*, 239244. [CrossRef] [PubMed]
41. Delanois, R.E.; Gwam, C.U.; Mohamed, N.; Khlopas, A.; Chughtai, M.; Malkani, A.L.; Mont, M.A. Midterm Outcomes of Revision Total Hip Arthroplasty With the Use of a Multihole Highly-Porous Titanium Shell. *J. Arthroplast.* **2017**, *32*, 2806–2809. [CrossRef]
42. Hosny, H.A.H.; El-Bakoury, A.; Srinivasan, S.C.M.; Yarlagadda, R.; Keenan, J. Tritanium Acetabular Cup in Revision Hip Replacement: A Six to Ten Years of Follow-Up Study. *J. Arthroplast.* **2018**, *33*, 2566–2570. [CrossRef] [PubMed]
43. Meneghini, R.M.; Meyer, C.; Buckley, C.A.; Hanssen, A.D.; Lewallen, D.G. Mechanical stability of novel highly porous metal acetabular components in revision total hip arthroplasty. *J. Arthroplast.* **2010**, *25*, 337–341. [CrossRef] [PubMed]
44. Shen, X.; Qin, Y.; Li, Y.; Tang, X.; Xiao, J. Trabecular metal versus non-trabecular metal acetabular components for acetabular revision surgery: A systematic review and meta-analysis. *Int. J. Surg.* **2022**, *100*, 106757. [CrossRef] [PubMed]

Disclaimer/Publisher's Note: The statements, opinions and data contained in all publications are solely those of the individual author(s) and contributor(s) and not of MDPI and/or the editor(s). MDPI and/or the editor(s) disclaim responsibility for any injury to people or property resulting from any ideas, methods, instructions or products referred to in the content.

MDPI AG
Grosspeteranlage 5
4052 Basel
Switzerland
Tel.: +41 61 683 77 34

Journal of Clinical Medicine Editorial Office
E-mail: jcm@mdpi.com
www.mdpi.com/journal/jcm

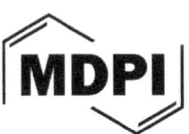

Disclaimer/Publisher's Note: The title and front matter of this reprint are at the discretion of the Guest Editor. The publisher is not responsible for their content or any associated concerns. The statements, opinions and data contained in all individual articles are solely those of the individual Editor and contributors and not of MDPI. MDPI disclaims responsibility for any injury to people or property resulting from any ideas, methods, instructions or products referred to in the content.

www.ingramcontent.com/pod-product-compliance
Lightning Source LLC
LaVergne TN
LVHW072252110526
838202LV00106B/2615